'Shielded':
A Diary of the Pandemic
2020–2023

Roger Davidson

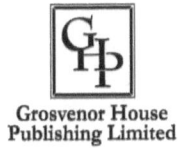

Grosvenor House
Publishing Limited

This book is published by
Grosvenor House Publishing Ltd
Link House
140 The Broadway, Tolworth, Surrey, KT6 7HT.
www.grosvenorhousepublishing.co.uk

A CIP record for this book
is available from the British Library

Paperback ISBN 978-1-80381-961-7
Hardback ISBN 978-1-80381-960-0
eBook ISBN 978-1-83615-009-1

For Mo

Contents

Preface

At some point in late December 2019, I alerted my wife, Mo, to a brief reference in the *Scotsman* to an outbreak of a new, severe acute respiratory coronavirus originating in Wuhan, China. I commented that the UK Government would do well to cease its preoccupation with the General Election and 'getting Brexit done' and prepare for what might become an existential threat. Subsequently, the World Health Organisation declared the spread of the virus as a Public Health Emergency of International Concern on 30th January 2020 and designated it as a pandemic on 11th March 2020. As a social historian I sensed that a period of dramatic change in our way of life was imminent and that this could best be captured for posterity by keeping a diary. Accordingly, I began to record our life with Covid-19 from 19th March 2020, just four days before a national lockdown was imposed.

Deciding on an end-date for the diary has been more problematic. Variants of Covid-19 are still circulating widely within the community. It is estimated that one in 24 or 2.5 million people in the UK are likely to have tested positive on 13 December 2023. In addition, evidence would suggest that over 1.5 million people are living with the legacy of long covid.

However, with the availability of vaccines, British society has learnt to live with the virus, and it is no longer perceived as an existential threat. A significant turning point came in May 2023 when the World Health Organisation announced that Covid-19 no longer constituted a 'global health emergency'. The recent proceedings of the Covid-19 Inquiry have also been indicative of a shift in public and political discourse towards a retrospective view of the pandemic and mark an appropriate endpoint for this diary.

There is a rapidly growing historiography addressing the origins and impact of the Covid-19 pandemic in Britain. Some commentators have focused on the virological and epidemiological aspects of the story and its implications for the social construction and influence of scientific and medical knowledge. Others have concentrated instead on the efforts of the policy community to contain the pandemic and the competing agendas of health and economic forces within Whitehall and Westminster. Meanwhile, medical historians have sought to locate Covid-19 within the context of past epidemic and pandemic diseases. Economic historians have explored the impact of quarantine measures past and present while historians of class, gender, and race, have focussed on the social disparities accentuated by the pandemic. Its impact on civil rights and restrictions has also drawn the attention of political and legal historians.

In addition, the pandemic has produced a range of research initiatives dedicated to recording and archiving the everyday lived experiences of people coping with the crisis since March 2020, often adding a sociological or even anthropological dimension to the historical narrative. Central to these initiatives has been the collection and analysis of diaries that provide a very special window into the mind-set of individuals faced with the threat of Covid-19 and its variants.

My diary, which records my responses to the pandemic from the first lockdown in March 2020, both as a social historian and a 'shielded' individual coping with Parkinson's Disease, will hopefully represent a valuable addition to the existing literature.

PART I

Lockdown
2020

19th March

Today, the full realisation of the meaning of 'self-isolation' hit home. We decided that until further notice we had to dispense with our cleaner. She, herself, is scrupulous in wearing gloves and keeping her distance, but she has family and care homes that she routinely interacts with, and she could easily be a vector without knowing it. However, we are going to keep paying her for the moment, partly as a retainer but more importantly to help in some small way to safeguarding her income. With the gardener the problem is less acute as for the most part he operates outside the house. But as some form of income support, we have signalled that we are happy to pay the going rate for a range of other tasks in the garden such as repainting the shed etc., albeit that these do not do justice to his skill set. People are being very solicitous, and I am receiving concerned queries about my condition from N on a regular basis; one today at 7.08! If nothing else, I hope this crisis drives people back into having proper telephone conversations rather than texting.

Yesterday, Parentline closed its volunteer help line – a very sad moment, not least because one fears that it will be a long time before it recommences, if at all, given the likely impact of the crisis on funding. The 'dream team' had already ceased to operate – I had given in my notice as a 'self-isolator', one of the team was quarantined at home because her family had unwisely taken a trip to Milan, and the other may still, as I write, be in lockdown in Tenerife.

Panic buying is still a problem and Mo is trying hard to arrange on-line delivery with a supermarket. If the reports are anything to go by, she will struggle as many of the distributors have no slots for weeks ahead. Meanwhile, problems with the supply of my Parkinson's medication are already kicking in. Fortunately, I always try to keep a 2–3week surplus, but I do not

2

fancy having to cope with my medication being interrupted. Brilliant reading of Hilary Mantel's third volume on Radio 4 – much better as an audio than as a read, if the critics are to be believed.

21st March

A visit yesterday to the bird hide at Musselburgh, a welcome break from the isolation of the house. Spectacular colours on the shelducks and vivid yellow flashes on the teal. But surreal trying to maintain distance from other birdwatchers and walkers. I am increasingly aware that even the country locations and bird reserves that I was looking forward to visiting are now crowded with everyone else who has self-isolated but seeking open air outlets.

The news from Italy is disastrous and if we mirror its experience, we are in for a frightening escalation in deaths from Covid-19 in Scotland. The Government is slowly but inexorably moving to some form of total lockdown. Yet, it is reluctant to police some form of containment, but given the continued disregard of advice by anti-social members of the community and the impending unravelling of the NHS as infected numbers spiral, 'lockdown' can only be a few days away. Certain at-risk groups are due to be contacted with a view to providing them with food and medication without having to leave their houses. I appear to be somewhere towards the bottom of the list, so I am still uncertain where I stand. Certainly, I am unhappy with Mo having to queue in shops and the pharmacy. We also need to ensure that the gardener and podiatrist do not present a possible risk of infection. There really is no end to the precautions that, ideally, we could take (for example, sanitising newspapers and post, all shopping, and any random deliveries). All we can do is use anti-viral liquid on surfaces, adhere to normal hygiene procedures and, most difficult of all, keep our hands away from our faces.

Today, we played our first game of scrabble – the first of many I suspect as we need to build in a variety of activities to mentally survive the next months. Already we feel disorientated by the absence of any commitments in our diaries and the lack of social contact – indeed I sometimes really struggle with remembering what day of the week it is.

24th March

The Government has, yesterday, at last introduced a form of lockdown. We are directed not to go out at all except for food shopping, limited exercise, and the procurement of urgent medical supplies. More things continue to unravel – problems of getting an MOT now garages are closing; the issue of whether we can risk visits from the podiatrist and whether the gardener can come in for his customary pee. Today we continued our ritual of de-cluttering the house by focusing on the hall cupboard – much in need of a coat of paint and some creative joinery. In a way we are finding this process therapeutic in the hope that, when we do get back to some semblance of normality, and commence the kitchen project, at least the rest of the house will be tidy and decluttered.

My Parkinson's is slowly getting worse I'm afraid and my feet are sticking dangerously at every turn. I shall persevere with the 8mg Ropinirole and try and steadily increase the dose over the next couple of months. Fortunately, I am good at sticking to an exercise routine and have been able to integrate my Pilates exercises into my own program. I do question how much longer I could have coped with Parentline, and certainly if the service was re-started, I would have to think very carefully if it was appropriate for me to continue. I do wonder though how charities are going to survive the crisis and whether Parentline has a future.

Received a very caring call from an old university friend concerned for our welfare. I shall miss meeting him in Stratford and sharing the Royal Shakespeare Theatre experience.

Meanwhile, my daughter, Hilary, seems to be in lockdown in Penicuik. There was talk of her being redeployed elsewhere in the NHS but thankfully nothing came of it. Martin, my son-in-law, is at the front line as a paramedic and has begun to deal with increasing numbers suspected of having the virus. The real worry is my grandson who appears to be disregarding government pleas and is hanging out with his friends. If he catches the virus, he will effectively commit Hilary and Martin to self-isolation at the cost of their health and contribution to the NHS.

2nd April

Second week of lockdown. Everything has become a perfect storm of anxieties and forebodings. Mo and I are managing well. In many ways, having spent a lifetime of solitary in the archives and behind my writing desk, being locked down is not too great a shock to my system. However, I do miss my Pilates for Parkinson's classes and above all the social milieu of Parentline. We have also missed our book group (Laura Cumming, *On Chapel Sands*) although, with the aid of Zoom, we are hoping to rectify this omission. Mo is suffering more from the social isolation as she is a natural socialiser. So far, she mainly compensates by endless conversations on the phone. Mentally I am fine and trying to keep mentally fit by doing the *Scotsman* crossword, playing scrabble with Mo, and doing some refereeing for academic articles on sexuality.

Sadly, my physical condition still deteriorates and my footwork has become so stilted that I am constantly at risk from falling. So, we have decided to access some music online and to do some dancing to try and improve my coordination. I do stick to a regular workout regime every day along with a rather 'Pythonesque' extended walk around the garden to maintain muscle tone. I am also increasing my doses of a new medication (Ropinirole) which may alleviate my symptoms. Ironically, the main warning on the information leaflet, previously brought to my attention by the Parkinson's nurse, is 'priapism and hypersexuality'.

We are interpreting lockdown fairly rigorously and now letting no-one into our house; necessitating a rather awkward call to our gardener to the effect that if he needs a pee, he will have to find a convenient spot in the garden! My only residual worry is that Mo is still having to shop occasionally for basic foods, although she has arranged for a regular delivery of fruit and vegetables, as well as a milk delivery. Until now, she has been okay with the situation, especially after the supermarkets got their act together with social distancing, but it remains a weak link in the lockdown and I am now insisting that we seek some local help.

To date I have not received the 'at extreme risk' letter but I have no intention of being a martyr to the sacred cause of 'herd immunity'. I strongly suspect that it is this epidemiological model that has led to the dangerous lack of testing facilities in the country, as I am sure Johnson's and Cummings's initial objective was to let the epidemic run its course, thus preserving the economy while at the same time focusing mortality on the elderly and most vulnerable citizens. Apart from the ethical issues raised by such an approach, it failed to recognise that such a model only worked if a vaccine was available. By the time our leaders took this on board there had been a fatal delay in ramping up our testing regime. Coupled with the ongoing failure to supply adequate PPE (personal protection equipment) to front-line medical staff, the Government is attracting increasing censure.

Curiously, Nicola Sturgeon has not made any comment on the mismatch between the English and Scottish mortality figures. On Monday through Tuesday 283 people died of the virus in the UK, whereas only 16 people died in Scotland. Hopefully there is some consolation to be drawn from this.

3rd April

Feeling vulnerable as I feel I am brewing something; the sort of nasal and throat discomfort that presages a cold, but God willing not more than that!

7th April

Considerable relief that, although I continued to feel under par, no Covid-19 symptoms developed; a reflection I think of the visceral fear this virus is spreading. Meanwhile, events have made the situation even more surreal. Not only has the Chief Medical Officer for Scotland had to resign for breaching her own self-isolation guidelines but Boris Johnson has succumbed further to the virus and is now in intensive care. There is a feeling that the Government's lockdown strategy is beginning to attract increasing scepticism and 'push back'. The policing of open spaces has drawn considerable criticism. Several European governments are now contemplating phased unlocking of certain sectors to try and avoid the total breakdown of their economies. In addition, a report has surfaced today suggesting that keeping children off school has minimal effect on infection spread. Government public briefing sessions are becoming increasingly vacuous with the same mantras about 'flattening the peak' and 'doing the right thing at the right time', with little insight into what the exit strategy from lockdown is going to be.

Today has been one of mixed fortunes. For the fourth time in six days Bella has been sick and dealing with the problem may not be easy in current circumstances. On the plus side, I managed to sit in the sun for 15 minutes and do 45 minutes gardening without any balance issues. Being close to the soil always energises me and dispels my health anxieties. Mo has been on the phone exploring whether any food delivery slots are available, but they are all occupied for the foreseeable future. I hope the Government does not impose any stricter lockdown because we could do without another senseless round of panic buying. Another boost to my ego – an approach from the *New York Times* to discuss the historical issues surrounding contact tracing and a request to referee an article for the *Transactions of the Royal College of Physicians of Scotland*. It is good to keep my academic skill sets honed.

14th April

The dreadful toll of the virus daily increases and it is now predicted that the UK will end with the worst death count (now well over 11,000) of any European country. Worryingly, there is growing concern that patients treated in intensive care units are being ruthlessly triaged, with those over 70 held back from any invasive treatment. The debate over the lack of personal protection equipment and community testing, and any vestige of contact tracing, continues apace. Meanwhile, the media is devoting increasing space to the torrid details of what it is like for both patients and medics in ICU's and the trauma and distress of relatives who cannot be with their dying family members.

Predictions for the future are dire with behavioural experts predicting that we shall have to significantly change our behaviours for the foreseeable future, such as not touching our faces or eyes, and that we will all need to wear masks. Spain and Italy are about to introduce a partial relaxation from lockdown, and it will be interesting to see whether this leads to further spikes in the number of people infected. Predictably, Trump is rejecting any criticisms of how the Covid crisis has been handled in the USA. He is now proclaiming that he alone can decide when the lockdown should occur, in contravention of the American Constitution and the coordinated plans already being framed by a range of State Governors.

16th April

In the last two days, the dire state of residents in care homes has been highlighted. In Scotland some 25% of deaths out of a total of 963 have been in care homes. The care community feel that they have been marginalised in the provision of PPE and testing. Particularly scandalous is the fact that hospitals have been offloading elderly patients to care homes without testing them. They therefore constitute a real risk of spreading infection that now exists in 45% of Scottish homes. Matt Hancock continues to evade pertinent questions at the daily briefings, uttering the same mantras each day about his 'ramping up' the provision of PPE and tests despite continuing evidence that there are critical shortages across the health and care systems. Meanwhile, it is becoming increasingly evident that the most vulnerable within the community, which probably includes me, will have to remain in 'shielded' lockdown for an unspecified period until a vaccine is available, as the virus will be in the community for many months, if not years, to come.

23rd April

Counting care home and community deaths as well as hospital deaths, the toll is now over 25,000 in the UK. Still the disconnection exists between the Government's claims over PPE and testing and the actual reality. More ominously, the Chief Medical Officer for England and Wales has predicted that social separation strategies will have to continue until effective treatments or vaccines are available, most probably on stream at the earliest next year. This has enormous implications for the economy and society and is a real 'reality check' for us all. Meanwhile, there are the first stirrings of 'push back' against the current lockdown regulations. Some Tory backbenchers are increasingly concerned to relax the restrictions for some sectors of the economy and there is anecdotal evidence that there is a gradual increase in travel by the public in contravention of the Government's guidelines.

On the home front the weather has been wonderful and sitting in the sun in the garden has been hugely healing. My exercises are going well, and I am feeling the benefit of some of the routines I learnt in the Pilates classes. Unfortunately, my 'festination' has worsened, and I am now suffering from repeated incidents of freezing. This means that, to avoid a fall, I am taking an unconscionable time to get from A to B. The Ropinirole tablets do not seem to have improved my condition at all, so I am retreating to an 8mg dose per day. Still no letter identifying me as in need of 'shielding' with priority for supermarket deliveries. Meanwhile, news that Hilary is going to be redeployed to help with testing in care homes. Worryingly, she does not share our concerns about the lack of PPE and her vulnerability as someone whose immune system has been severely compromised over the years.

Parentline's new procedures seem to be up and running with calltakers operating from home. Sadly, if the forecasts of the virologists and epidemiologists are correct, the shift room will not be operative again until next year. Hopefully, Parentline will see that, realistically, if they are going to retain all their volunteers, they need to employ more of us to operate from home, subject to further training.

Router flashing orange for the last 12 hours and no access to the internet. I have tried switching a number of plugs on and off but to no avail. Sadly, it looks as though I will have to try and get some advice from BT. Usually, I can use our neighbour, but this is no longer possible with lockdown. Just one more problem created by Covid-19!

28th April

I am writing this while I listen to the daily whitewash briefing defending the Government's achievements. It has all the hallmarks of 'fake speech': the same old mantras of 'following the science' and doing 'the right thing at the right time' without any acknowledgement that most other countries have been far more effective in closing borders and undertaking testing and contact tracing. Not surprisingly, the revelation that there have been very significant numbers of deaths in care homes has attracted increasing attention.

Today, I have at last received notification that I am in the 'shielded' group of individuals at the highest risk of serious/ mortal harm from the virus. It comes with a directive that I should stay completely locked down until at least the 6th of June! This enables me to have priority in the allocation of an online food order and distribution slot from the supermarkets which will reduce the need for Mo to run the gauntlet of shopping precincts.

Increasingly, I am seeking relief from the incessant round of intrusive interviews with bereaved families and endless documentaries on the cause and course of Covid-19. Instead, I am listening to the classical CDs that I bought with part of my retirement present. Today, Barber's Adagio for Strings which I originally heard as the soundtrack to *Platoon*. Very moving and a possible choice for any cremation, should services be possible sometime in the future.

29th April

I am increasingly concerned at the military rhetoric employed by the Government. Clearly, Cummings et al are intent on covering up their incompetence by trying to create a false sense of wartime 'we are all in it together' social unity. In reality, the growing evidence of failures to equip front-line medical and distribution staff with adequate protection against the virus is producing the first real signs of social discontent. As one ICU consultant observed, they can label us 'heroes' because it then goes some way to justify our deaths. A sinister alteration to the official briefing in England is the introduction of questions from the public at the expense of the more forensic questions posed by the media. In addition, the membership and recommendations of SAGE (Scientific Advisory Group for Emergencies) is coming under the spotlight. There is growing concern that Cummings has attended meetings and that certain recent decisions, such as the failure to participate in European PPE initiatives, have been inappropriately shaped by political agendas more to do with Brexit than Covid-19. The fact that, in the face of all the current mayhem, the Government is determined to stick to the existing deadline for transition arrangements for Brexit says it all!

A better day health-wise; more fluid movement and less festination. This enabled me to garden with much more confidence. I just wish I knew what made the difference from one day to the next. Off now to see if Mo is up for a dancing session to improve my balance.

30th April

Finally, the Government has come clean about the extra numbers of Covid-19 deaths in care homes and the community: some 4,000 extra deaths that brings the total to over 27,000, with the UK now on target to record more deaths than any other European country. I suspect it is no coincidence that the additional deaths were announced on the same day that Boris's baby was delivered. One can just hear Cummings arguing that it was a good day to bury bad news. Meanwhile, criticism is growing from NHS trusts that the Government lacks any clear strategy in its testing policy and that key workers are still not being adequately tested. Other 'grey' voices are beginning to question what appears to be a discriminatory approach to the elderly, both in the egregious neglect of the care homes and in the debilitating lifestyles required of those over 70 in lockdown and 'shielded'.

The Covid-19 crisis is truly transformative in its effects on social life. To date I have resisted any form of online or telephone banking, and indeed never used an ATM machine in my life. But, as I cannot now personally go to the bank, I have been forced to move with the times, albeit very, very slowly.

1st May

The Government's much-vaunted target of 100,000 tests per day appears to have been achieved and Johnson is arguing that this will form the basis of a gradual release from lockdown.

However, it is not evident that we have any strategy for processing the test data. Ideally, we need to follow up with systematic contact tracing, followed by the isolation and treatment of the vectors identified. Clearly, we have yet to create an army of tracers, and once more we are well behind the curve. For meaningful tracing to be achieved we first need to get the number of infected within the community well down and this will take weeks, if not months. The current problems all stem from the failure to impose stringent controls and to introduce widespread testing and compulsory isolation at the beginning which, the current spin of Health Ministers notwithstanding, was a consequence of the early adherence of policy makers to a 'herd immunity' model. Indecision in late February and March, coupled with the scandalous lack of stockpiled PPE, has cost us dearly. Yesterday, in a rather breathless attempt to regain centre stage in the discourse surrounding Covid-19, Boris announced in his first public appearance at the daily press briefings that we were 'past the peak'; words that may well come back to haunt him!

I wonder where (and how) we will all be a year from now! If we survive the virus, how far will the Parkinson's disease have reduced my quality of life still further? How many of our close friends will still be with us? And will the kitchen renovation ever have been completed?!

2nd May

The focus of the debate surrounding the pandemic is now shifting to how the test data can be used to facilitate an incremental relaxation of current controls. The medical advisers are focused on using the data to establish the level of R (viral reproductive rate) in the community so that they can identify sectors/regions/ social groups that might be released from lockdown with least effect on the numbers infected and requiring hospital treatment. In order to upgrade the capacity for contact tracing one proposal being seriously considered is that the Government will issue an app. to all those with mobile phones in the community as a means of locating centres of infection. Quite apart from the fact that you need about a 50–60% take-up to make this viable, there are serious ethical issues relating to privacy that need to be addressed. Meanwhile, various forms of treatment to reduce the trauma of intensive care for Covid-19 patients are being tested in the leading pharmaceutical laboratories, including the use of blood plasma from those who were previously tested as positive for the virus and have subsequently recovered.

In the USA, Trump's behaviour is outrageous and even his allies in the media, such as *Fox News*, are starting to distance themselves from his more unhinged utterances. At one press conference he was heard to mutter that a possible medical option might be to inject patients with a disinfectant. Meanwhile, he is clearly driven by the need to try and recover the US economy before the forthcoming election whatever the collateral damage to the nation's health. Consequently, he has criticised State governors who, fearing a second spike in infections, have adopted a cautious approach to the relaxation of lockdown conditions. Indeed, Trump is now giving more than tacit support to the views of (frequently armed) protestors demanding the return of free movement and economic activity.

3rd May

Our 23rd wedding anniversary. Fond memories of quaffing champagne in the garden of the Selkirk Arms with Chris and Paul and our surprise interlopers, Martin and Hatty. With lockdown, there is no opportunity to go out for a nice meal or to visit friends.

However, we skyped Uddingston and Canada. I fear that online chats are going to be the main form of communication for the foreseeable future. I wonder whether they will shape relationships in a different way. So much of our social behaviour and customs is likely to be permanently altered by the pandemic.

10th May

The debate over Covid-19 drags on with little evidence that the Government have a clear strategy for testing. They are experimenting with a contact tracing app. on the Isle of Wight, but it appears to me that, without an army of trained contact tracers in the field, no clear picture of the level and location of the infection will emerge. Meanwhile, the objectivity and membership of SAGE has been questioned, underpinned by the growing awareness of the media and policy community that science is in fact socially constructed and that members of the Committee, and their modelling, may well be driven by various competing intellectual and professional agendas, as it was formerly with HIV/AIDS. The sociologists of scientific knowledge will have rich pickings when they come to review this crisis.

Relations between Nicola Sturgeon and Boris Johnson appear to be cooling further. Boris wants to grandstand the gradual unlocking process, however minimal it may be, with the threat that the key policy mantra of 'stay at home, protect the NHS and save lives' will be dropped. Sturgeon resents learning about this via the media and considers such a move to be potentially disastrous, not least because she is advised that the R factor is higher in Scotland and perilously close to 1. I fear that the outcome of the debate over the next fortnight will be a revised strategy that very gradually enables the economy to re-start but coupled with an even more rigorous lockdown for the vulnerable and 'shielded', including my good self.

PS I was gratified to see that several political commentators share my belief that Cummings was the leading advocate of the misguided early 'eugenic' strategy of aiming for 'herd immunity'.

11th May

Boris has now begun to outline his so-called 'road map' for releasing lockdown in England. However, the presentation of this initiative has been so badly handled that it has created widespread confusion. The 'stay at home' mantra has been replaced with 'stay alert' – a vague and ambiguous message. Workers have been asked to return to work provided safety measures are in place but told not to use public transport. It is unclear what employment rights they have if they refuse to work when faced with a work situation that is clearly not Covid proof. Boris has also declared that reception classes and primary 6 classes should return to school by the end of May, but the teachers' unions are adamant that, as things stand, it will be impossible to ensure these children adhere to social distancing. They also rightly demand to know just how far this is actually based on solid epidemiological intelligence. Most irresponsible of all, it is proposed that in England people are now to be permitted to travel any distance for the purposes of exercising. This will inevitably lead to a mass exodus to the coast or countryside, thus compromising the health and slim hospital facilities of these areas. The fact that, in Scotland, Nicola Sturgeon is sticking to the old mantra of 'stay at home', demanding that Boris's new guidelines not be circulated north of the Border, and continuing to restrict recreational travel to a minimum, further adds to the confusion. The policing of mobility guidelines that vary across the

United Kingdom will be a nightmare. Bizarrely, only now has the Government decided to regulate arrivals at British airports from abroad by imposing on them a mandatory two-week self-isolation regime, a measure that should have been introduced at the very start of the crisis. Even more bizarrely, these new checks will not apply to arrivals from France and Ireland! It is clear the political consensus that characterised the early weeks of Covid policymaking is now fracturing at a rate off knots.

12th May

Predictably, the regional variance in the guidelines for movement has created a great deal of confusion. While in England one is now permitted to visit garden centres, you still cannot visit more than one of your parents! In Scotland, neither is permissible. That workers returning to their employment in England can maintain social distancing in public transport has proved delusory. Meanwhile, the media has been eager to demystify the Government's claims over testing. Their claim to have attained 100,000 tests a day is spurious as they are counting in test sets posted out but not necessarily completed. In reality, the figure is probably well under 50,000.

My Parkinson's is sadly deteriorating. My walking now lacks fluidity, and I am constantly freezing or juddering with the ever-present fear of falling. The addition of Ropinirole to my extensive collection of medications does not seem to have had any effect but I might try upping the dosage again. The other major problem is the behaviour of my bladder. At times it displays an embarrassingly acute urgency and seems to be impacted by my bowel movements. I can live with this for the moment, but it will become a very inhibiting factor if and when we are ever set free from lockdown. I can still just do some gardening, especially cleaning the drive and watering the flowerbeds. I wonder whether I will still be able to do even these routine tasks in 2021?

Bella remains a constant joy; so affectionate and biddable. We are truly blessed to have her.

16th May

You could not make it up! The Government's Covid-19 policy is like a Mad Hatter's Tea Party. Boris is full of vacuous bluster and clearly has no grasp of detail. Meanwhile, according to one wit, Matt Hancock is suffering from 'repetitive floundering syndrome'. Their initiatives appear to be off the cuff and full of inconsistencies. People may travel as far as they want in England for the sake of exercise, but not in Scotland and Wales. While employees are being encouraged to travel to work in London by car, the congestion charge has been reintroduced. While the Government is pushing for a selective return to schooling on 1st June, there is no hard evidence as to how far children can transmit the virus and no credible guidelines that will ensure social distancing in classes. The right-wing press is putting outrageous pressure on the teaching unions to allow teachers 'to be heroes', and to step up to the Covid challenge, no doubt with the inevitable outcome of deaths within the profession. Today, concern was being expressed that the R factor was rising, but nevertheless quintessentially middle-class pursuits – golf, tennis, garden centres etc – are being unlocked in England. All along, the politicians have been covering their backs by claiming they were just 'following the science' but increasingly it is evident that it was, and still is, the political agenda that is shaping, or more accurately misshaping, health initiatives. In addition, testing is still haphazard and far from providing a firm basis for policymaking.

Meanwhile, Trump is excelling himself in oafish ignorance and spite, dismissing his pandemic experts and claiming to be a new Darth Vader who will conquer the virus with a massive injection of funded research on a level with the development of the nuclear bomb. Most sinister of all is the revelation that he has secretly been attempting to do deals with the pharmaceuticals so that the USA will have first access to any vaccine and control of the patents!

More positive developments, however, on the home front. We have decided to designate the living room as an activity area during the day. Yesterday, Mo installed a firestick so we can now access *You Tube*. We have begun to exercise along with *Dance for Parkinson's*, put online by members of the Royal Ballet Company. In addition, I dusted off my guitar and spent a blissful hour jamming along to Muddy Waters, fantasising that I was Eric Clapton (or Eric Clapped Out as Mo would put it). There is also a possibility of participating in an on-line training course on domestic abuse run by Children First which would be a welcome addition to my counselling skills.

Today, the podiatrist called. She is the one exception to our lockdown policy and the first person across the threshold in 7 weeks! We all wore masks and she sanitised all her equipment, and we located the sessions in the conservatory to increase the airflow. Both Mo and I have toenail issues and it made no sense to ignore our regular appointments if we subsequently had to seek emergency treatment. For me, with my balance problems, the health of my feet is paramount. Sadly, the presence of ambulances next door together with the protective gear now being worn by our neighbour's carers (including her son) suggests she may have tested positive for Covid-19.

Watered the garden again today as we have had virtually no rain over the last eight weeks. The beds are looking fabulous and Mo thinks it is the drop in air pollution that is making the colours more vivid. Certainly, the garden is a huge consolation during lockdown.

17th May

Sadly, our next-door neighbour has died. We all stood on our doorsteps as a mark of respect as the funeral service's cars left. It makes the threat of this virus feel all too real!

20th May

It appears that in recent weeks some 45% of Covid-19 deaths in Scotland have been in care homes. This makes it all the more nauseating to hear politicians claim that from the start the Government placed 'a protective ring' around the care home sector. It is such spin that generates an ever-increasing distrust in policymakers. The medical experts and politicians are already at loggerheads as to who was responsible for the decision to abandon systematic and comprehensive testing in late March; as a result of which, current initiatives, such as the possible return of children to school in England and the 'unlocking' of certain leisure and employment activities, appear devoid of scientific basis.

22nd May

Yesterday, Nicola Sturgeon introduced 'Scotland's Route Map through and out of the Crisis' detailing various conditional stages for an 'unlocking' process. Unfortunately, her guidelines for the 'shielded' will only be issued in the next couple of weeks. We are therefore left with a very difficult decision as to whether or not, and when, we reactivate the kitchen renovation project.

For the moment, we have rescheduled the work for late September in the hope that, by then, decanting to Portobello won't constitute such a risk. Still battling to get a food delivery slot. Apparently, Midlothian shielding group can only forward requests to the supermarkets and thereafter it is up to the supermarkets to respond.

I am very conscious of my 'festination' varying from day to day. It is evident that tiredness is a major factor and that clear-headedness is vital for my mobility.

28th May

An eventful week on the Covid-19 front dominated by the furore surrounding Dominic Cummings's breach of the lockdown rules and his arrogant press briefing in the gardens of 10 Downing Street. There have been strong calls for his resignation from the public and politicians, including a sizeable group of Tory backbenchers. However, clearly Boris is totally dependent on him and refuses to sack him. Throughout, there has been no word of contrition. Significantly, Boris's ratings in various polls have dipped dramatically in the last fortnight. Last night's live performance of Boris before the Commons' Liaison Committee (the first time he has deigned to attend it since last May!) has only underlined his inadequacies as a leader. He waffled and huffed, avoided answering the questions, and had no command of the details of policymaking. It was like watching an ill-prepared fourth-former in a school debate. It should be added that he still does not look well, and one wonders whether he is 'fit for purpose' – certainly not on yesterday's showing.

Today sees the launch of the Government's much vaunted 'Test and Trace' strategy designed to lock down individual vectors rather than the whole community. This is a huge gamble. There is no comprehensive testing programme firmly in place and the contact tracers have had minimal training. Moreover, the initiative presumes that everyone who is informed out of the blue that they have been in close proximity to some anonymous person testing positive for Covid-19 will comply with the request to isolate for 14 days, whether or not they, themselves, are seropositive. As Jack Dee would say: 'Good luck with that!'.

Meanwhile, on the home front, the splendid weather is enabling us to make the best of our wonderful garden. The ballet exercises for Parkinson's are now on our regular schedule as is my guitar jamming. Our book group has reconvened, using Zoom. Parentline has also been in contact. They are trialling various scenarios involving either the shift room or taking web chats at home. Given my 'shielded' status and my imperfect keyboard and computer skills (especially with my tremor) I have declined for the moment from participating. It may sadly be, after 18 years, the end of my help-line career: we will see!

Later today, Sturgeon is due to update us on the next phase of Scotland's handling of Covid-19. While I anticipate that certain aspects of lockdown will be relaxed, I fear that the 'shielded' may be the exception and asked to continue in total isolation.

29th May

As I feared, the 'shielded' are not included in the latest 'easing from lockdown' guidelines. Instead, we are left with a vague promise to deal with the 'shielded' in the next two weeks and meanwhile to stick to our strict isolation. Ironically, I have only just received authorisation from the DVLA for an extension to my driving license. As it expires by the end of next January,

I have already lost a third of the extension year! Meanwhile, the videos by Janey Godley, with her voice-over of Nicola, continue to provide enormous entertainment.

30th May

Another brilliant, sunny day which seems out of kilter with the times, given that confirmed deaths from Covid-19 is now just shy of 40,000 and the calculated excess deaths over the last three months compared with the five-year average is north of 60,000! Worryingly, several medical members of the Government's advisory group, SAGE, have now broken ranks and argued that the impending relaxation of Covid-19 guidelines is premature given that the R factor is still very near 1 and the 'test, trace and isolate' process is still being created. In their view, the decision to relax guidelines has been based more on political than strictly scientific considerations. In the view of some in the media Johnson insisted on announcing the 'Test and Trace' initiative at an earlier date than was expected in order to try and divert the growing political fall-out from Cummings's perambulations. Sir David King, former Chief Scientific Advisor to the UK Government, has also aired his misgivings. He predicts the possibility of a second wave of infection if the Government ends lockdown prematurely. In his opinion, there is still a dangerous level of infection in the community, and he points out that the level of infections now is no less than it was when lockdown was first authorised. Meanwhile, the failure of the much-hyped app.-driven contact tracing trial on the Isle of Wight (Matt Hancock's supposed 'game changer') has been assiduously ignored in official briefings.

31st May

Overnight, and without reference to any credible 'evidence base', the Government has relaxed the guidelines for the 'shielded' in England. As with the other relaxations, many senior medical experts, including several members of SAGE and the Association of Directors of Public Health, are concerned that the whole situation will unravel and a fresh spike in infections materialise. In Scotland, the position of the 'shielded' remains unchanged for now. Nicola Sturgeon is right to be cautious given that, according to the latest estimates of Covid-19-related per capita deaths, Scotland has one of the worst, if not THE worst record!

Long phone call with Hilary today. She is now being redeployed to contact tracing. She says that contrary to the exaggerated claims of the Scottish executive, the tracing system in Scotland is a shambles. She was given just one hour's training, mainly taken up with general information about the pandemic but no focused advice on the tracing process and forms. Apparently, even the basic paperwork for the tracing has not yet been signed off by Health Protection Scotland. And yet her trainer implied that she would be starting work on Monday!

1st June

Here we are in the eleventh week of lockdown. I am increasingly spending time listening to music and find it very therapeutic. Many years ago, in 2007, I purchased out of part of my retirement present from my university department a range of classical CDs for us to play in our caravan at Sandgreen. In the event, we played very few of them and it is only now that we are settling down to appreciate them properly. If nothing else, it has underlined my dreadful ignorance of the history of music, composers, and musicians.

3rd June

A perfect storm at the heart of the USA: race oppression, Covid-19, and summer heat leading to widespread vandalism and rioting; further inflamed by a psychotic President who sees an opportunity to win votes by advocating armed suppression of the rioters, without a word of empathy for the black victim murdered in cold blood by the police in Minneapolis. On a less apocalyptic scale, a perfect storm also in the UK: increasing distrust in the Government's handling of the pandemic with daily exposés of the continuing inadequacies in the testing and tracing processes, stark predictions by the business and transport sectors of an impending economic melt-down with associated catastrophic levels of unemployment, and the imminent prospect of a no-deal Brexit with all the disruption and uncertainty that will entail!

4th June

A typically full day mixing Royal Ballet exercises, some watering of the garden, a period of reading for the book group [Emily Maitlis, *Airhead* – an excellent read], and an hour listening to classical music [a wonderful rendition of Tchaikovsky's Violin Concerto by Nigel Kennedy] before settling down to view the daily vacuous Covid-19 performance from Westminster.

7th June

We are entering the 12th week of 'shielded' lockdown. The total of all tested and confirmed Covid-19 deaths is now above 40,000 and total excess deaths over the period compared with a 5-year average is estimated to be c.60,000. The Westminster Government is introducing various exceptions to the lockdown designed to try and avoid total economic disaster but based on unconvincing/absent medical evidence. The scientific community is increasingly at odds with this liberalisation of society and fear a second wave of the epidemic will be triggered. The politicians argue that with a comprehensive 'test, trace and isolate' system in place, together with a 2-week quarantine imposed on all arriving at British borders, they will be able to locate local hotspots of infection and suppress them. Sadly, evidence from Health Boards and from testers and tracers, suggests that this system is still very much a 'work in progress'.

Meanwhile, in Scotland, Nicola's caution in maintaining rigid controls appears to be validated by the number of people breaching the travel guidelines last weekend. However, two issues continue to throw doubt on her handling of the pandemic. First, the fact that the Scottish Executive failed to publicise and act upon the Scottish 'ground zero' of infection – at a Nike conference in Edinburgh in February. Secondly, it has recently been revealed that, in 2018, a simulated exercise was undertaken in Scotland based on the MERS outbreak which revealed the vital need in any future pandemic for an adequate stock of PPE and ample facilities for testing and tracing, together with a responsive strategic plan; recommendations that were clearly ignored.

An emotional day on the domestic front. Family trauma dating back to the 1970s re-surfaced with a vengeance and forced me to face some of my demons yet again. I felt like someone out of a Stephen Poliakoff play, viewing an old wedding photograph in which each character had a story to tell.

9th June

As I anticipated, Nicola Sturgeon announced yesterday that those who are 'shielding' could expect to say in lockdown 'until at least the end of July'. There might be some relaxation of the exercise guidelines in her review of 18th June, but this would be conditional on the infection rate remaining low. I felt very deflated at the news as I had hoped we could now at least travel a little for some walking/scootering. The thought of another 10 weeks lockdown is depressing and will come perilously close to the time we had scheduled for the kitchen renovations and our decamp to Portobello. The gap between the English and Scottish guidelines appears to be daily widening and, if it gets any wider, we might even have to have 'border controls'! The fact that the Government has had to do a U turn on opening schools to all primary classes in England, given the logistical issues involved and the opposition of the teaching unions and many parents, suggests that Nicola has a more realistic and evidence-based grasp of the appropriate scale and timing for our release from lockdown.

Government policymakers blithely believe that they can now set the economy free from many aspects of Covid-19 controls and that they can rely on their new 'test, trace and isolate' procedures to dampen down any consequent local upsurges in infection. It is a hugely risky strategy that I think, rightly, Nicola is not at this point prepared to take. The high mortality rate in Scottish care homes has clearly had a profound effect on her and she is not prepared to witness a further culling of the 'shielded' by releasing Scottish controls prematurely.

This morning was dominated by computer glitches, with the hub going all the colours of the rainbow except blue! Despite my best efforts, the router continued to flash orange at me, having flirted with green and purple! Thankfully, a call to BT solved the problem but the episode reinforced my awareness of how dependent we are on broadband technology for almost every aspect of our lives.

10th June

A disastrous morning trying to sort the broadband connection again. The usual Mad Hatter's Tea Party routine with Open Reach. Earliest appointment early July and advised that their engineer would not come into the house during lockdown. After resetting computer to another free BT network on the advice of a neighbour, suddenly the magic blue reappeared on the router and my original network connections restored! [Later: computer down again!]

Interestingly, Radio 4's *More or Less* programme revealed that one of the reasons for the belated decision to lockdown in March, with a consequent loss of lives, was due to inaccurate advice given to SAGE by experts modelling the pandemic. Apparently, they significantly underestimated the rate of increase in the number of infections, leading to undue complacency on the part of Boris Johnson and the Cabinet. Meanwhile, Richard Horton, Editor-in-Chief of the *Lancet* has also launched a vitriolic attack on the Government's scientific advisers, dismissing the daily Corvid-19 briefings as a 'betrayal of science'. He is incensed by the two scientists standing 'like altar boys and girls either side of the hapless minister du jour'. In his view, 'our scientific community has become the public relations wing of a government that has abjectly failed to respond to this pandemic'. Sociologists of scientific knowledge will have a field day with the Covid-19 story in years to come!

12th June

The Government is coming under increasing attack for its handling of the pandemic. There is mounting evidence that, at the high point of the epidemic in February and early March, some 25,000 patients were released from hospitals into care homes without being tested for Covid-19. There is also incredulity at the claims being made at briefings that the 'test-trace-isolate' procedure is operating well. Anecdotal evidence suggests that many contact tracers are sitting idle and many of those identified in the tracing process refusing to isolate. There continues to be no sign of the so-called 'game changing' app.!

Yesterday, I received my new instructions from the Chief Medical Officer [CMO] for Scotland requiring me to stay put until the end of July. There may be some relaxation after 18th June of the restrictions on outside exercise, but only if the infection rates in Scotland are deemed low enough. Some of the instructions are hopelessly unrealistic. I am supposed to stay 2 metres away from anyone else in the house, including Mo, and to keep 2 metres away from anyone I live with if and when I am permitted to go out for a walk!! One is left wondering what planet some of these medical experts live on.

Mo is suffering from a slight sore throat today. In normal circumstances this would just be annoying, but at the moment it raises fearful issues. I pray that my next entries augur well!

14th June

Thankfully, Mo feels much better. Yesterday, we had to compromise our 'shielded' status a little to allow the BT engineer to deal with our internet problems. In the event, we managed to keep our distance and the engineer was careful to sanitise all the surfaces he had touched. As a result of his efforts, we now have a broadband speed of over 30!

The Sunday papers have extensive coverage of the unravelling of consensus within the policy community. Even among the scientific advisers there is growing discord. Given that the level of viral reproduction within the community is still dangerously close to 1, albeit with regional variations, the epidemiologists, along with the CMO for England, are reluctant to endorse any significant relaxation of the lockdown restrictions, such as the opening of non-essential retail outlets now scheduled by Boris Johnson for tomorrow. Meanwhile, the behavioural scientists advising SAGE are stressing the psychological damage that continued lockdown will inflict and the urgent need for schooling and employment to return to some semblance of normality.

Now a week into my higher dose of Ropinirole. I cannot detect any improvement in my movements but I will stick on a 12mg dose for a couple more weeks. In normal times, I would be keen to have some bloods taken to check that my cocktail of medications is not doing any actual damage, but a routine visit to the phlebotomist would not be a sensible risk at the moment. The garden is looking fabulous, and whether or not it is the weather or the Covid-19-induced clean air, the roses are stunning in a variety of vibrant colours.

17th June

Interestingly, yesterday's official briefing was delivered by the Foreign Secretary without the usual entourage of expert advisers. Rumour has it that the CMO and Chief Scientific Adviser have become increasingly disenchanted with being used as a 'shield' for political accountability. The fig-leaf of 'following the science', used by the Cabinet to cover their naked incompetence, had threatened to compromise the professional integrity of medical experts, especially when they were expected to answer politically charged questions from the public and the media at the daily briefings.

The weather today is overcast and oppressive and it will be a blessed relief when we get some clear air and sunlight. Gradually making progress listening to our classical CDs. A high point has been the cello performances of Jacqueline du Pré, playing the cello concertos of Dvorak, Haydn and Elgar.

20th June

Amid the customary grandiloquent claims, many of the Covid-19 restrictions in England are being lifted over the next few weeks. The Government claims there has been a significant fall in the level of infection within the community. It is claimed that the infection is no longer increasing exponentially [so-called level 4 alert] but merely circulating within the community [level 3] and that this is sufficient to take the risk of opening most retail outlets, including hospitality venues with outdoor spaces, and setting a timetable for the return of children to school by September. This rather dramatic shift in policy possibly reflects growing unease in Westminster at the loss of public confidence in Johnson's ability to provide decisive leadership. Moreover, at a time when the national deficit is approaching the net value of GDP, the Chancellor is understandably arguing for an early release from lockdown, backed by the business, leisure and entertainment sectors who face widespread failures and redundancies. The pressure to restore schooling and further education as soon as possible has been compounded by the concerns of paediatricians and psychologists at the collateral damage to mental health being inflicted by the lockdown. Yet, one is left wondering just how robust the epidemiological justification is for these departures. The 'test-trace-isolate' machinery is still not fit for purpose, not least because the tracing app., hyped by Matt Hancock, was found to be incompatible with I-Phones and a replacement is now not anticipated until sometime in the autumn!

As for Scotland, Nicola Sturgeon continues to play a cautious hand. Even though, in terms of per capita Covid-19 mortality, Scotland stands third in the world [!], She also is under enormous pressure to restore employment and education and, subject to the level of infection continuing to decline, she is slowly navigating her exit from lockdown. Sadly, there is little release from my 'shielded' restrictions and depressingly little to show for 13 weeks of confinement. According to my official text, 'I can now go out for a walk, wheel, run or cycle, if I stay 2 metres away from other people' (a bazaar request, given that Mo appears to be included in 'everyone') and only travel for a few miles'. I can also choose to meet people from one other household outdoors each day' and 'take part in other non-contact outdoor leisure activities in my local area.' It is clear that many people are now interpreting some of the guidelines (such as the 5-mile limit for non-essential journeys) very liberally and I suspect that from now on we will rely on our own risk management and common sense. So come Monday, some friends from Dalkeith will join us in the garden and celebrate our blessed, if partial, release from house arrest!

22nd June

Glorious piece by Rod Liddle in the *Sunday Times* skewering the competency of Matt Hancock. To quote: *'The lockdown delight in our household is Hancock's Half Hour, in which the health secretary stands before the cameras and explains how he's screwed everything up yet again. We settle around the television with pizza and nacho chips, ready to fall about laughing. There is something in his expression-immense but terribly misplaced self-regard, which is always in danger of teetering into petulance-that makes the viewing so poignant, as well as hilarious. A middle manager from a carpet warehouse suddenly put in charge of whether we should be allowed to continue existing or not. His "hi-tech, made-in-Britain, state-of-the-art, Bluetooth Covid-testing app" riff is an enormous crowd-pleaser.'*

Felt distinctly unwell this morning first thing; mainly feeling faint and clammy. An extra 30 minutes in bed with some tea and a biscuit seemed to aid recovery. I suspect it has to do with my medication and at the end of this week I intend to rein back my Ropinirole to 10mg to see if that makes any difference. I may also build in some brief rest periods into my day.

24th June

Major relaxations of the lockdown in both England and Scotland with varying dates but generally Scotland is initiating changes a little later than Westminster. This will effectively mean that, in addition to the previous release of retail outlets, the leisure and hospitality sectors can re-open, subject to appropriate hygiene and distancing procedures being in place. Boris has also lowered the distancing requirements from 2 metres in an effort to enable venues to be financially viable. Nicola is still taking advice on the self-distancing restrictions. Masks are now mandatory on transport and in all venues, although for the moment the Government is pursuing a 'light touch' on its enforcement.

Significantly, the CMOs are continuing to stress that the virus will be with us for a while yet and that there will almost certainly be a second wave of infection in the winter. In many ways the Government still has not got an exit strategy as such. In the absence of a vaccine, given that only about 35% of the population has some level of immunity from Covid-19, the only effective option would be to ensure that the testing and tracing procedures were sufficiently robust and decentralised. This might enable the rapid suppression of local spikes of infection, and the gradual total elimination of the disease. Evidence would suggest that the contact tracing is still inadequate and that, without a tracing app., a large proportion of potential contacts are being missed. Meanwhile, the Government appears to have at last woken up to the fact that quarantine requirements on all inward-bound travellers are increasingly a nonsense given that many European countries have a much lower level of infection than the UK. The time for stringent quarantine controls is long past and they do little more than cripple our tourist and aviation industries.

Bad fall last night has left me very shaky and lacking in confidence. One moment I was upright in the kitchen and then, in a flash I was spinning out of control onto the floor. Fortunately, it all happened so quickly that I did not have time to put my hand out. A blessing also that I fell through the kitchen doorway so that my head did not collide with any hard surfaces. Above all, thankful that Mo was close to hand. I suspect tiredness and the side effects of my medication were to blame. Maybe, in addition to cutting back on the Ropinirole, I will experiment again with using the walker indoors; another watershed in my condition, but so be it!

Ps. A sign of the times was witnessing on Zoom yesterday 7 very respectable members of our book group discussing the relative merits of various urinary devices designed to enable greater mobility during the lockdown, given the closure of all public and retail outlet toilets.

29th June

General confusion and chaos have ensued following Boris's premature announcement of wide-ranging relaxations of Covid-19 restrictions on July 4th – our so-called 'Covid Independence Day'! Not only have the health guidelines for England and the remainder of the UK now diverged but fuelled by the dangerously up-beat narrative of Johnson, together with the temporary heatwave, many people are now openly congregating in large numbers on beaches, at beauty spots, and at organised raves, with little regard for social spacing.

30th June

100th day since lockdown. Already the loosening of controls in England is proving problematic with Leicester being re-locked down to address a spike of infection in the area (an early example of Boris's new 'whack-a-mole' strategy! You really could not make it up) How it is going to be policed is another question! Meanwhile, Scotland continues to diverge from England in important aspects of Covid-19 policy. According to Nicola Sturgeon's last public briefing session, whereas Boris is prepared to tolerate a certain level of infection in the general population as long as the NHS is not overwhelmed, in Scotland Nicola is actively seeking Covid's elimination. Consequently, she is not relaxing quarantine restrictions on overseas visitors coming into the country and has hinted that imposing controls at the English Border remains an option.

The usual mix of activities today; weeding the driveway, some reading, a few exercises, and further attempts to learn basic scales for my guitar. Footwork and balance are bad and I have to be careful not to tire my legs out as this leaves me very fixed and unstable by the evening. Mo has established a good routine of online delivery from Morrison's, although, despite my repeated efforts, none of the supermarkets has ever contacted us since lockdown. Watching a lot of short sketches performed by various theatre companies during Covid-19 to sustain the arts through this crisis; hugely creative and talented. Also gripped by *Cardinal*, a gritty and often brutal detective series from Canada: marvellous photography, albeit a stomach-churning plot. Its depiction of the icy wastes in Algonquin Bay really brings home the desolate existence northern Canadians must endure.

1st July

A forensic examination on Radio 4's 'More or Less' of the mistakes made in handling Covid-19. In particular, it highlighted the failure in March to impose controls at the airports. In the period leading up to lockdown, some 16 million people entered the UK, predominantly from Western Europe where the virus was already reaching its peak. Of these, only 263 were tested and quarantined. This complacency was compounded by the mistaken belief that the UK was a month behind other European countries in the spread of infection when in fact we were only about 10 days behind. While Boris and his advisers thought infection numbers were only doubling every 10 days, they were in fact doubling every 4–5 days. It is estimated that by 5th March some 50,000 people in the UK were infected. Many experts now believe that this failure to lockdown earlier with proper testing and tracing cost some tens of thousands of lives and explains why the UK Covid-19 mortality rates have been so high compared with other countries.

Another area of mounting disquiet has been the sclerotic performance of Public Health England. It appears that at every stage of the crisis it has insisted on a centralised system of provision and controls and ignored all the existing expertise and resources of local laboratories, regional public health directorates, environmental health officials, and GPs. It has also failed to provide local health officials with real time test and trace data that might enable them to anticipate the need for further lockdowns.

Mo and I tackled another Royal Ballet class for Parkinson's today. As per the previous class, much was lost in translation, but we both felt energised.

8th July

Today, the Scottish Health Secretary is due to issue new guidelines for the 'shielded'. Hopefully, this may mean we can have a more active social life. In the last week, the debate surrounding Covid-19 has become increasingly heated and chaotic. There are several worrying features of recent developments that stand out for me. First, in many countries, including England, unlocking social venues has led to a spike in infections and a consequent need for re-locking. Secondly, evidence suggests that nearly 80% of patients in the UK who have tested positive have suffered no symptoms. This means that there are a vast number of people out there in the community who appear to be perfectly healthy but who can infect others with fatal results.

Meanwhile, the Scottish Health Secretary, who should have resigned many moons ago, has admitted that over the last month there has been no follow-up checks on incoming travellers quarantined at the airports due to issues of security clearance with the Home Office. It really beggar's belief!

I have had time in the last months to reflect more and more on my life. Until now, I had always considered myself to have been very fortunate not to have been involved in any war or pandemic (other than a brief visit for Andrew's wedding in Canada during an outbreak of SARS). I even narrowly missed having to endure National Service. It is then ironic, that in my final years, I should be faced with my first real existential challenge (not counting Parkinson's and a stroke) so late in life.

9th July

New guidelines issued yesterday made very little difference to my regime. Shielding is to be retained at least until the end of July. I can now see more people at one time (2 households rather than 1 each day) provided I self-distance and remain outside. If absolutely necessary, I can also use the toilet at another house that I am visiting. No mention was made of travel restrictions, but it appears that other than local travel is still discouraged. Ironically, the major change highlighted by the Scottish Health Secretary was that I no longer needed to distance myself from 'the people I live with'! Just how they think Mo and I could have ever complied with such unreal expectations, we will never know!

11th July

The world has certainly gone mad! Yesterday, it was announced that the previous disaster of a Transport Minister, Chris 'failing' Grayling, is destined to become the Chair of the Intelligence and Security Committee, viewed as a key advisory committee of British governance. [Subsequently, after what was described as 'a very English coup', another Tory was voted in as Chair with the support of Labour and the SNP. Johnson was incandescent and the new Chair was promptly suspended from the parliamentary party. Given that the raison d'etre of the Committee is to provide an independent oversight, this episode was one more instance of the Government's determination to emasculate existing processes designed to hold it accountable].

14th July

Today was the first occasion that we were able use the scooter this year. A lovely smooth, tarmacked path from Innerleithen towards Peebles. Somewhat alarmed at the operating light going into flash mode, which needs checking. It was a tonic to be out in the open air again, albeit with bladder constraints. Tomorrow, a whole range of more liberating guidelines are scheduled for Scotland, but as Nicola has stressed this is going to be a very risky few weeks. Sadly, some experts are already predicting a torrid winter with flu and Covid-19 and the possibility of 100,000 deaths! Coupled with Brexit this is a daunting prospect.

17th July

The UK Government's handling of the Covid-19 crisis continues to unravel. The Chief Scientific Adviser has openly challenged Johnson's new policy of encouraging people back to work before the level of new infections has been properly brought under control. Whereas Nicola has a clear strategy of eliminating the virus before total relaxation of Covid restrictions, Boris appears to want to jettison the 'stay at home and save lives' mantra for a more populist, 'get back to work for the economy' approach that conflicts with public health priorities and threatens a second wave of infections. Meanwhile, the 'test and trace' procedures continue to be plagued by shortcomings. Some of the commissioned test kits have proved ineffectual and there is no sign of any 'game-changing' app. on the horizon. Certainly, there is clear evidence that local authorities are not being fed the prompt and detailed information on Covid contacts that is needed for any so-called 'whack-a-mole' approach to sporadic spikes in infection around the country.

18th July

Boris has now raised the stakes by shifting the responsibility for getting the workforce 'back to work' to employers from 1 August and by expressing his anticipation that we may be a significant way to returning to 'some form of normality' by Christmas; a view clearly not shared by the Chief Medical Adviser.

22nd July

Went yesterday to Gosford Estate. A lovely run on the scooter around the ponds (policies), with heron and greylag geese in abundance. As usual, bladder problems were a downer, but I am gradually learning to literally 'go with the flow' and just use a urine bottle in the lee of the car door. Tremor in the legs and hands make for an exciting performance! Recently, my mobility and balance has certainly deteriorated, and I can do less and less gardening. I find it especially sad that I can no longer deadhead all the roses properly. I am increasingly conscious of my life inexorably narrowing (and sadly Mo's as well as my carer). My response is to try and sustain as wide a range of interests and activities within the home as possible.

On my birthday we were joined by friends, Gerry and Susan, for a distanced glass of champagne and an Indian take-away in the conservatory. They are relatively new friends – lively and engaging and thoroughly rewarding to be with. Gerry, talented soul that he is, having won 'Master Chef' twice, gave me his painting of the Dalkeith Water Tower, which they had transformed into a residence some years ago. Mo did sterling work organising the occasion and ensuring that I had a really enjoyable 78th birthday.

28th July

Some of the previous restrictions on the 'shielded' have now been relaxed and the First Minister has even suggested that by the beginning of August the 'shielded' program might even be suspended if the infection levels remain as they are. I can now meet with more people out of doors and meet with up to 8 people indoors from two other households, subject to keeping 2 metres away from others and avoiding crowded places. I can also go into shops and travel on public transport wearing a face covering and sit outside at pubs and restaurants. My first reaction is ambivalent. In many ways, now a more liberal regime has been introduced for the general public, there is even more of a risk of encountering an asymptomatic Covid-19 sufferer. This is especially so given that, despite the grandiloquent claims of Hancock and Johnson, we lack a trace and contact system that permits health authorities and the public to know in real time where infection spikes are present.

I received a wonderfully supportive and encouraging message from my supervisor at Parentline. It is clear they are happy to have me back and to facilitate any renewal of my call taking. I just hope I can rise to the challenge. My main problem is the increase in my tremor and agitation which in turn exacerbates my bladder issues. I really need to discuss all this with my GP but I fear that she will be fully occupied with Covid-related work.

2nd August

A very confusing time. On the one hand, Nicola has now suspended the 'shielding' process but, on the other, in the North of England Boris's 'whack a mole' policy is in full swing with much of the recent relaxation of controls reversed. Daily recorded deaths from Covid-19 are still approaching 100 and the overall mortality is heading steadily towards my initial prediction of 50,000. Increasingly, robust international comparisons show the UK as having performed worst in controlling the pandemic with Scotland faring little better. There has been a significant retreat from Boris's earlier inflated prognostications of a return to some form of normality by Christmas. Instead, the politicians and the experts are predicting the likelihood of a second 'wave' of Covid-19 infection coupled with the annual cycle of winter flu. Increasingly the experts are framing the narrative of the next few weeks as a trade-off between social and medical priorities; the price of letting children go back to school being the closure of pubs and other leisure and hospitality venues where infection is more likely to spike.

We are trying to get out more using the Berlingo and scooter and beginning to have friends round to the garden, and sometimes conservatory, while preserving social distancing. I had a wonderful Zoom meeting with the Parentline 'dream team' – so bonding! I have now established with my supervisor, that I will make a firm decision after the kitchen renovations are complete in October. She is fine with this and hugely supportive of me coming back and renewing my call-taking. I just hope my coordination, agitation and tremor improve before then, not to mention my bowel and dribbling!

6th August

An unremitting stream of bad news: escalating business closures and redundancies, unprecedented falls in dividends that underpin pension schemes, and resurgence in the level of Covid-19 infections. Experts are predicting that, in the absence of a comprehensive and effective system of 'test, trace and isolate', the opening of schools and the associated return to employment will lead to a fresh wave of infection in the autumn that might be at least twice as acute as the first onset of the disease. Worryingly, evidence suggests that the follow up from tracing is targeting only about 50% of contacts and that there is still no rigorous policing of contacts to ensure that they are self-isolating. Meanwhile, other health experts are predicting that additional deaths through the neglect of non-Covid conditions during the last few months may be greater even than those resulting from the pandemic.

The weather has been very changeable and lacking in real warmth. The prospect of coping with Covid-19 anxieties in the winter months is daunting. My mobility continues to be a major worry with the need for me to be vigilant every second of the day, especially when I am turning. I have lost a great deal of physical confidence and I wonder how I shall fare if and when I recommence my help-line commitments. On the plus side, we have now identified a few venues suitable for extended use of the scooter and this opens up the prospect of more ventures out and even some birdwatching.

12th August

The news continues to cast a bleak shadow over our lives. Today, the economy has officially been designated as in a recession; a fall of 22% in GNP between April and June (a worse performance than any other developed economy). High unemployment in the autumn is widely being predicted. Meanwhile, the scientific and medical communities are seeking to learn the lessons of the first wave of Covid-19 in anticipation of a second wave in the winter. It is increasingly clear that some 30,000 lives could have been saved if we had previously developed stocks of PPE and robust testing equipment and procedures in preparation for a pandemic, and the Government had introduced lockdown at least one week earlier.

Spectacular lightning and thunder last night with torrential rain. Fortunately, our cul-de-sac seems to drain very effectively but elsewhere there have been a spate of landslips, including one that derailed a Glasgow–Aberdeen train at Stonehaven, causing fatalities.

My walking is especially dire today; long periods of freezing and lack of mental and physical confidence. It is difficult to know just what makes my coordination vary from day to day. Perhaps it is the heat as today is probably the hottest yet.

13th August

Managed to do some gardening today but my legs gave out after about an hour and my tremor made it increasingly difficult to operate the garden tools. I suppose I just need to reconcile myself to doing a little bit of weeding each day.

16th August

Mixed feelings today. I cannot help thinking about the damage Covid-19 has done to teenagers, compounded by the insensitive and inequitable handling of the allocation of school grades by the Government and education authorities. It must feel like an utter betrayal of all they have worked for, especially as this is a cohort that has had to live through lockdown. More generally, but no less damaging, in a very real sense they have been deprived of their 'rite of passage' usually associated with the completion of one's schooldays. Goodness knows what legacy has been left of mental health problems for the future!

On a more positive note, the Edinburgh International Book Festival has responded to Covid-19 by delivering its programme online. Last night, we enjoyed excellent presentations by Val McDermid and Maggie O'Farrell, both giving fascinating insights into their writing and wider views on current events. In some ways, this is an ideal format for me as it enables me to access my favourite cultural event without having to travel into Edinburgh. We also welcomed the fact that it cuts out the often irrelevant and self-referential questions from the audience that bedevilled the live performances.

20th August

Once again you could not make it up. Hancock's latest 'game-changer' amidst the pandemic is to integrate Public Health England with NHS Test and Trace in an allegedly new National Institute for Health Protection. To compound the crass stupidity of reorganising Health Service agencies in the midst of coping with Covid-19, he has appointed the erstwhile head of NHS Test and Trace,

Dido Harding, to direct the new venture; the very person who presided over the previous failure to develop an effective tracing app. for the UK, having had a previous disastrous record at TalkTalk. It is not perhaps a coincidence that her husband is a major fund-raiser for the Tory Party! A cynic would see this as a further effort of the Government to offload blame for their mistakes onto Public Health England and onto the very experts who they formerly used as a shield in their public briefings.

Sadly, the incidence of new infections in Scotland is rising again including some outbreaks in schools. At today's Scottish briefing, Nicola was not prepared to acknowledge that Scotland could advance into a further stage of exit from lockdown. Rather, she emphasised the need for continued working from home where possible for non-essential occupations, and for stronger police powers to enforce guidelines relating to distancing and tracing. First Minister's question time also reflected the growing concerns of parents and the teaching unions that, unless more stringent action was taken in schools to ensure masking and distancing, the attempt to restart education would unravel.

Another excellent presentation from the Book Festival: Jim Naughtie speaking about US politics. He predicts that if Trump fears he will lose, all hell will break loose, and he will refuse to relinquish the post of President and exploit all the divisiveness that he has nurtured in American society.

26th August

A dismal day after stormy weather. Scottish Gas are now here for the third time of asking to fix the boiler which has begun to sound like a jet engine taking off. I am keeping my fingers crossed, as it is imperative that we get it fixed (hopefully not replaced) before our kitchen renovations. The Covid-19 situation continues to be a mess. The schools have gone back but there is every prospect that there will be outbreaks of infection and the reinstatement of local restrictions. Meanwhile, Holyrood and Westminster are continuing to diverge over the use of face coverings in schools, a debate that has exposed major disagreements within the policy community and educational establishment. Most scandalous is the enduring inadequacies in the test and trace system, with some people in Scotland being directed to testing stations hundreds of miles away, including Northern Ireland!

It all feels like a perfect storm, with little sign of any remission from the virus in the short to medium term, with a no-deal Brexit on the horizon, with the worrying prospect of Trump being re-elected this year and IndyRef2 validated in next year's Scottish elections, and with my mobility, tremor, and bladder issues increasingly eroding my quality of life. After the kitchen is completed, we must agree on a more rewarding life strategy. My role will primarily be to enjoy home and garden comforts with the minimum of stress and an appropriate array of aids and therapies, while Mo should be free to develop her social and cultural life without having to wait on my tortuous progress! That way both of us can live a more fulfilling life.

31st August

I have decided that the time has come to be more proactive with respect to medical and paramedical issues and arrange for some bloods to be taken, for a dental check- up, for an appointment with the optician and physiotherapist, and some discussion with my GP over my aortic aneurysm.

The Sunday columnists rightly portray the SNP's grandiose claims for the Scottish economy and its ability to cope with independence as 'beyond delusional'. It is estimated that Scotland's deficit will soar to 28% of economic output, with a dramatic fall in tax receipts from North Sea oil and gas, the continuing economic repercussions of Covid-19, and a no-deal Brexit 'piling uncertainty and disruption on a fragile economy' [David Smith, *Sunday Times*].

4th September

Disturbing news from Nicola Sturgeon that the R factor for Covid-19 in Scotland may now be as high as 1.4, which raises the possibility of another wave of infections and another lockdown for the 'shielded'. Worryingly, an increasing number of school children are proving positive. There is a continuing failure to provide coordinated, competent, and accessible 'test, trace and isolate' procedures. Without these, any policy of 'back to school' or 'back to work' runs the danger of spikes in infection getting out of control. Meanwhile, we have the ludicrous situation of travel-related quarantine restrictions varying from one part of the UK to another: yet another issue that could be more readily addressed by universal testing and tracing of those arriving at airports. Moreover, if the process was extended to all residents of retirement homes and their carers the cruel isolation of the very elderly and/or demented from their relatives could be relaxed.

Talked to the Parkinson's nurse yesterday on the phone in lieu of my six-monthly appointment. Clearly, the nature of the beast is such that there is no specific proven palliative for my 'freezing of gait', recognised as a symptom of mid-stage Parkinson's. We have decided that, for the moment, I will increase the Ropinirole slowly up to the 24mg originally suggested by my consultant. Meanwhile, in line with my resolution to be more pro-active in addressing medical issues, I have arranged for bloods to be taken to check that my cocktail of medications has done no serious harm.

9th September

Government very much on the back foot as Covid-19 numbers escalate again. All of England is now subject to strict limits on the number of people who can socialise (the somewhat unfortunately named 'Rule of Six'), and on the range of permissible venues. Some towns in Wales and the North of England have been locked down again. There continues to be a lack of accessible testing facilities and the countries from which travellers have to isolate on arrival in the UK fluctuates day by day and differs between the various parts of the nation.

The Government's Covid-19 speak has created a whole new vocabulary:

'We are following the Science' (we intend to offload accountability for the failures in addressing the virus onto our advisers)

'We are doubling down' (we are hideously behind in preparing for this pandemic and now panicking)

'Ramping Up' (ditto, often just to attain impressive numbers without regard to quality and delivery).

'We wrapped our arms around' (we had to come up with some cosy phrase to try and excuse our egregious neglect of care homes)

'Granular approach' (an expression designed to make a policy of whack-a -mole less risible).

'Nuanced' (government speak for supposedly a more flexible and sophisticated approach to the pandemic, made possible by an illusory grasp of the data).

'Doing the right thing at the right time' (exercising post-hoc rationalisation for every error along the way).

'Oven Ready' (a half-baked policy that is based on wildly deluded claims of the extent to which Covid preparations have progressed).

10th September

Johnson has really excelled himself today. Having belatedly woken up to the fact that testing and tracing is the key to controlling the pandemic, his response to the 'uptick' (another new word to add to Covid-19-speak) in infections is to propose 'Operation Moonshot', intended to deliver by the end of the year 10 million tests per day at a cost estimated at 100 billion pounds, equivalent to three quarters of the annual cost of NHS England. Unsurprisingly, given the failure to establish even a modest testing service to date, his proposal has met with widespread incredulity. I just wonder whether Cummings and Johnson have flown this kite as a means of distracting attention from the political fall-out from their Internal Market Bill that openly contravenes the Northern Ireland Protocol that was a central plank of the legally binding Brexit Withdrawal Agreement under which Britain left the European Union last January. This is a flagrant violation of International Law, and one that might seriously endanger the Good Friday Agreement, as well as erode the devolved powers of Holyrood.

Meanwhile, Nicola has also re-introduced fresh limits in Scotland on socialising (no more than 6 people in 2 households) in response to a significant rise in the level of new infections and a suspected rise in the R rate to 1.5. In addition, a new tracing app. has been launched in Scotland, but it remains to be seen if this is any more effective than the abortive efforts south of the Border.

13th September

Hectic progress yesterday with Hilary and Martin making a wonderful input to the process of preparing for the kitchen/dining room renovation. My only contribution was just to stay out of the way which I managed only too gratefully. Two comments on the radio have stood out for me; that, while missing military conscription, my generation is in a way privileged to be involved in one of the most challenging episodes of the last 100 years, and instead of thinking of myself as *dis*abled I should see myself as *differently* abled, and thus shift to a more positive mindset about my ability still to offer something to others.

16th September

Preparing for our move to Portobello while the kitchen/dining room is being renovated as one room. Sadly, I can be of little use other than to avoid falling and to keep out of hospital! The Covid-19 news is not good. The level of new infections is rising steeply and medical experts are predicting a second wave to the pandemic. The failure to get on top of the virus is increasingly attributed by the experts to the inadequacies of the test and trace system. With the increased demand for tests from hospitals and care homes as well as from parents and employees now the schools have recommenced and more and more furloughed workers are returning to work, the testing system cannot cope. The problem is exacerbated on the supply side by the shortage of laboratory staff to process the swabs. Many of the skilled medical technicians who had previously volunteered to manage the testing centres have returned to their academic posts. The failure to use the previous expertise of the local public health authorities in favour of central initiatives has been an added constraint. Evidence also suggests that there is a significant failure to isolate on the part of the contacts of those who are found to be seropositive.

In yet another U turn, the Government today is now putting severe restrictions on who can apply for a test, with the NHS and care homes having priority. So much for Johnson's much vaunted 'Moonshot'!

My mobility is poor today, but we have acquired a new indoor walking device with trays that hopefully will enable me to move more easily about the house. It will also enable me to carry several items at a time from one room to another. My dribbling due to excess saliva is becoming a real pain, but on the recommendation of the Parkinson's nurse I am about to use a mouth spray designed to address this inelegant problem. (I note that Billy Connolly shares this indignity, although he has the benefit of using it for his comedy routine!). I started the day with 50 minutes of upper body exercises, and this has energised me. In addition, 10 circuits of the garden which I would dearly love to build on before the winter closes in. I hate being so dependant, but I suppose I have to be realistic and focus on what I can still do. Interestingly, the other day I broke into floods of tears playing along to Dire Straits – a sort of suppressed primal scream moment when all my defences were down. It was in one sense cathartic but also an insight into how near the surface my demons have become.

I must stay positive.

17th September

The Government's attempt to control outbreaks of Covid-19 appears to be unravelling at a rate of knots, largely because the testing system is still not fit for purpose. Today, semi-lockdown with curfews have been imposed on north-east England. We are hoping and praying that we don't suffer the same fate once the kitchen/dining room renovation begins next Monday! It will be interesting to experience two weeks in Portobello and to witness at first-hand how Covid-19-compliant the shops and seafront are. Meanwhile, Johnson excels himself by adding to the pandemic lexicon with his evocation to 'squash this sombrero' [a new variant, God help us, of 'whack a mole'] in the hope of suppressing a second wave of infection and securing some vestige of Christmas.

19th September

Boris Johnson has declared that we are now entering a second wave of the pandemic. The local lockdowns do not seem to have been sufficient to contain the spread of infection in the general community. The number testing positive for Covid-19 virus is doubling every eight days and it is predicted by the experts that this will have repercussions for ICU intakes in the next weeks with an associated rise in the number of deaths. As I write, large swathes of Northern England and the Midlands are now under new stringent guidelines with respect to socialising and hospitality venues. It is anticipated that London will follow. In Scotland, many areas in the West are under new restrictions and Nicola Sturgeon has given notice of a 'circuit breaker' lockdown coming into force next week. The R factor across the UK is now estimated to be between 1.1 and 1.4. Many medical experts are of the opinion that we must now accept that Covid-19 is now endemic in the UK and, rather than trying to suppress it, we should protect the most vulnerable while allowing education and employment to re-start and permitting the virus to run its course without recourse to repeated lockdowns. I suppose, in essence, this is akin to the 'herd immunity' approach that some leading experts were advocating way back in March. Their view is that a policy of trying to eradicate the disease is only viable if you have an effective vaccine. Others are less certain that it is possible to isolate the vulnerable indefinitely and that, with the winter flu virus approaching, the NHS will again be in danger of being overwhelmed. They argue that the priority is for policymakers to get a grip on the 'test, trace, and isolate' system that will enable a more nuanced and effective approach to managing the pandemic.

Off to Portobello today. Mo looks exhausted after days of packing and project managing. Thankfully, Hilary has come on board to help, including assisting Mo to take Bella to the cattery. I have focused on keeping out of the way!

20th September (Portobello)

Unremittingly bad news in the Sunday papers. The UK is recorded as having the 5th largest death toll in the world from Covid-19. It is estimated that between March and September there have been 65,000 excess deaths due to the pandemic compared with the 5-year average. It is also predicted that in 2020 the UK economy will contract by over 10% and that unemployment will be over 8% by the end of the year.

21st September

Monday Covid-19 briefings anticipate a need for more drastic action. It is predicted by the CMO and CSO that unless behaviour changes, there will be 50,000 new infected persons by the end of September and 200 deaths a day by mid-October. The number of infected in the community is doubling every 7–8 days and the Covid-19 alert has now been raised to 4, meaning that the level of the pandemic is on the verge of rising exponentially. As only around 8% of the population appear to have been affected, the 'herd immunity' approach is a non-starter. It also ignores the after-effects on those who suffer from the disease (the so-called 'long-Covid-19') and the strong possibility that sufferers may become re-infected.

Today, we reconnoitered Portobello for possible parking places from which to use the scooter. Very much a learning process. Many possibilities were closed off by illegal/ inconsiderate parking. In addition, we realised that we cannot park parallel to the kerb as there is the danger that, if another person parks close behind, we cannot reload the scooter. I need to obtain an appropriate disability poster for the rear window. The weather was gorgeous – blue skies and azure blue sea. From the seawall, spotted turnstones and Arctic terns.

The work has now started at Eskbank and Mo is in regular contact with the gang. They say they are making good progress but need to firm up on the number and position of the radiators. This evening we watched a new series on ageing relationships called 'US'. Brilliant acting by Tom Hollander, albeit some of the comedy was a little too close to home. [Unfulfilled wife to somewhat autistic, inflexible husband: "Are you ever going to be spontaneous?" Response: "I hadn't planned to be"].

22nd September

A major step-change in the UK's battle against the pandemic. Nationwide controls have now been imposed. In Scotland, we can no longer visit other homes or host visitors ourselves. Goodness knows how this will affect Mo using family to clear up after the kitchen/dining room upgrade! Mo liaising again with the kitchen team as well as caring for me. Not surprisingly, she is very tired and very stressed. However, we parked for a sea-view along from Joppa (spotted arctic tern, turnstone, common gull, redshank, bar-tailed godwit, oyster catcher). Later, a Zoom session with the Book Group. As always, lovely to see them and gossip, but sadly, the pandemic preoccupied discussion and marginalised the more enriching and cultural aspects of our lives.

Also noteworthy is the intrusion of the SNP's IndyRef2 agenda into Nicola's presentations. She has heavily hinted that her ability to adopt a more supportive approach to sectors of the Scottish economy and to compensate those on low incomes forced to isolate by 'test and trace' were in part due to her dependence on the dictates of Westminster and Exchequer funding.

25th September

A lazy morning reading Hilary Mantel's *Wolf Hall*. Mo back at Eskbank project managing. Some ominous developments in the Covid-19 situation. The levels of infection in Scotland are now the highest since the virus first arrived. There are serious outbreaks across the university sector giving rise to speculation that, in a worst-case scenario, students might not be permitted to go home at Christmas. In addition, there is evidence that less than 20% of those identified through 'test and trace' procedures self-isolate. All very depressing as the prospect of Covid-19 overhanging the rest of my life becomes ever more real.

27th September

Nearly a quarter of the UK population is now under special restrictions and an increasing number of medical experts and commentators are predicting a second lockdown before long.

28th September

The media is full of the 'Second Wave' of the pandemic and the consequences for civil society. An abortive trip to the Gosford Park Estate which appears to have closed to visitors again. Instead, we enjoyed a brief get-together with Jack at Longniddry Bents. Very strange not to be able to greet him with a hug! Strangely, for me, a highlight of the week was the possible sighting of a lesser redpoll and a grey wagtail!

30th September

The work on the house appears to be nearing completion. Happily, Mo now seems more relaxed after a period of extreme stress, given all the decisions she has had to make over the kitchen; stress exacerbated by my own limitations and the restrictions on securing friendly advice due to Covid-19. It has been a daunting project, but the trades team have been superb and always gone the extra mile for us. In addition, Hilary and Martin and the neighbours have been wonderfully supportive.

The US election debate says it all. Trump has trashed the level of public discourse in the States and these debates vividly reflect the lack of integrity and moral compass in American politics. Meanwhile, as I type, PMQs is underway, and Boris is displaying the same proclivity to denigrate his opponents and rely on a series of vacuous mantras and disclaimers. Once again, news of government initiatives brings to mind the Mad Hatter's Tea Party. It is reported that Priti Patel has seriously considered a scheme to decant asylum seekers to Ascension Island, some 4,000 miles away!

2nd October

Tomorrow, we return to Eskbank and the new kitchen/dining room. With minor reservations, this has been an excellent bolt hole, but I am beginning to go stir-crazy without our conservatory and garden. Our hopes for frequenting Portobello seafront have been largely unrealised due to parking issues, the lack of toilets and the press of visitors. Certainly, in the future, Longniddry Bents seems a better bet.

The Covid-19 situation is dire. Major pronouncements by both Boris and Nicola that there is an imminent danger of the virus again becoming out of control and that, if new restrictions are not adhered to, another national lockdown might be unavoidable. The latest figures seem to indicate that we are back where we were in mid-May.

News today that Trump has Covid-19. One's immediate reaction is that this is no more than his just deserts. However, I am concerned that Trump will merely turn this to his advantage; perhaps by re-scheduling the election and enabling his campaign to refresh its strategy, or more likely by representing himself as the brave warrior who risked his life by mixing with the American people and who conquered the virus.

5th October (Eskbank)

Now back at home and the new kitchen/dining room is spectacular. With help from Hilary and Martin, Mo has worked furiously to restore the house to some order. As a result, we shall be collecting Bella well before her scheduled uplift. The project has been a huge success and a worthy testimony to Mo's sustained efforts throughout, and the brilliant teamwork and skill of the tradesmen. We were so lucky to have it completed before either a second total lockdown was imposed or one member of the team had to isolate. Undertaking the project inevitably had a Covid-19 risk factor given the number of people working in a closed environment. However, the current trend in the UK infection rates and the probable delay in the availability of any vaccine would suggest that we would have had to wait forever for a window of opportunity.

As I write, the news media are analysing the reckless behaviour of Trump that has led to the White House becoming an epicentre of infection, with the President essentially a super-spreader! Mixed in with the febrile pre-election atmosphere in the US this is fast creating an existential challenge to American civil society.

9th October

The new kitchen/dining room looks outstanding and under Mo's aesthetic gaze is beginning to feel homely. Bella thankfully seems to have survived her stay in the cattery. She has been quite needy but very affectionate. Mo is very tired and run-down after all her project managing and a bout of cystitis has laid her temporarily low, but a course of antibiotics appears to be doing the trick.

The Covid-19 news is dismal. The level of infection in the Scottish population is said to be doubling every 9 days with a similar escalation in numbers requiring hospitalisation. In response, the Scottish executive has re-introduced stringent controls on the hospitality sector across the Central Belt. Although 'shielding' has not been renewed, official guidelines for the vulnerable sections of society echo the advice previously given in March. I fear a new lockdown is imminent; so ironic at a time when Mo now has a lovely dining room in which to entertain! Hopefully, at the very least we can drive to see the autumn colours, but even then we would be breaching the travel advice now in place.

12th October

A further warning from the BMA and senior medical advisers that the number of Covid-19 infections are 'spiralling out of control' and that these will translate in the weeks to come into a consequent increase in hospital admissions, in demands on ICUs, and in deaths. The social politics surrounding local restrictions are becoming increasingly fractious and for the first time since the onset of the pandemic in March there appears to be a real push-back against government directives that appear incoherent and lacking in scientific justification. The 'herd immunity' school of thought continues to challenge the 'lockdown' approach of the Government.

The kitchen/dining room is proving a great success and has moved the centre of gravity of the house during the day away from the living room. A nice mix of activities this weekend; guitar practice, scrabble, exercise, reading Hilary Mantel, preparing for next week's book group and the University's Gender and Sexuality Zoom seminar.

I am upping my Ropinirole to 12 mg today and starting to take a sub-lingual spray for my drooling. It is clear from my discussion with the GP last week that I am unlikely to obtain routine blood tests or a scan for my aortic aneurism in the near future. The most that I am likely to receive is the flu jab, which directly contradicts the previous message of the CMOs that the NHS was still open for non-Covid-19 treatments.

14th October

Dismal news to greet the day! As long as 3 weeks ago, it appears that SAGE advised the Government that nothing less than a circuit-breaking total lockdown on cities in Northern England would avert a fresh wave of infections with disastrous consequences. Moreover, the CMO for England has expressed grave doubts that the new tiered system of local and regional directives will suffice to control the pandemic. It remains to be seen how closely Scotland will remain aligned with developments south of the Border. Another depressing announcement that there is some tangible evidence that Covid-19 does not necessarily accord future immunity to those suffering the disease. Finally, as I feared, Trump has politicised his illness and recovery and is presenting himself as a hero that conquered the disease and 'took one for America'. One can only hope that he has a serious relapse – not fatal but enough to take the smug narcissistic smirk off his face!

16th October

Another bad Covid-19 day. The social consensus that marked the initial efforts to stem the spread of the virus has broken down. Whole swathes of the UK are now under special measures in semi-lockdown but there is no alignment between the devolved administrations. Some civic authorities such as Andy Burnham, Mayor of Greater Manchester, are resisting the diktats of Westminster. More seriously, senior scientific advisers are not convinced that the restrictions currently being imposed will serve to contain the second wave and that within 2–3 weeks we will be back where we were in April with the NHS toiling to cope. The continued failure of the 'test, trace and isolation' process to provide a robust picture of the pandemic makes this all the more probable. It is estimated that as few as 18% of those testing positive are self-isolating. As with the provision of PPE, 'test and trace' was fatally flawed from the start in that instead of using existing expertise, the process was contracted out to firms owned by Tory cronies who lacked clinical expertise and any experience of public health epidemics. All this against the backdrop of an imminent no-deal Brexit and a violent and divisive US election makes for a perfect storm. The news today that Russia is circulating misinformation about the Oxford vaccine trials only adds one more layer to the bleak picture facing us.

On a more cheerful note, the kitchen/dining room is proving a great success and it has quickly become the social hub of the home. It is a pleasure to have such spacious and functional facilities. On Wednesday, I participated on Zoom in a seminar run by the Gender and Sexuality Research Group at the University. It was a real buzz to be in the academic arena again and be able to do so from home.

22nd October

The Covid-19 news is dire. Yesterday, the number of recorded deaths was as high as those reported in early May! In response, Nicola is about to launch a 5-tier pandemic control plan designed to match the degree of social regulation to local levels of infection.

It remains to be seen how this will impact the previously 'shielded' members of the community. However, two more rewarding features of yesterday. Although strictly against the guidelines, we drove down to Innerleithen to see the autumn tree colours and give ourselves a much-needed break from the house. Later, I managed to solve the problem of how we continue to support M. given that we are not supposed to have outsiders in the house and we can no longer use the garden to entertain visitors. I managed somehow to set up Skype for us and we had our first Skype call.

23rd October

Today, Nicola has set out her 5-tiered Covid-19 strategy designed to deploy a calibrated set of controls according to regional and local variances in the incidence of positive cases. I have still to digest the details but what really sets the tone of the coming months is the observation of the Scottish Clinical Director that we would be deluded to think that we will be able to have a 'normal' yuletide. In his words, we should anticipate a 'digital Christmas'. The R rate in Scotland is thought by the experts to now be between 1.2 and 1.5.

27th October

A mixed day. Some ominous news that the number of deaths in the UK from Covid-19 had risen [in the new parlance of the Government's health spokesmen, 'an uptick'] by 60% in the last week. Also, more evidence that the immunity gained by those having been infected might be short-lived.

A relaxing and invigorating call to my old college friend, Alan, a retired judge. We spent a happy hour recalling our college days and colleagues. He is politically the polar opposite of Mo and me, but curiously we have a very fond relationship. As always, I think it is about mutual respect which is so lacking in civil society today.

30th October

Still awaiting the final decision on which Covid-19 tier we are going to be allocated to. Unfortunately, Dalkeith is relatively high up the infection league table, possibly due to the number of care homes in the area. News this morning that there is evidence that a significant proportion of the infections in recent months have been due to a variant Coronavirus originating in Spain and brought back by holidaymakers who were rarely tested and quarantined on their return. If this proves to be true, it is yet another example of the egregious failure to control our borders during the pandemic.

I had a long Zoom [I hour 50 minutes!] with the Parentline 'dream team' last night. It was lovely to hear them both in full flood. We are so lucky to have formed such a bond. I also got an update on the state of play at Parentline. Clearly, they have been doing sterling work during the pandemic and have emerged very much as the one fully active branch of Children First. I hope this will lead to some form of permanent funding for the service which is long overdue. The Zoom session confirmed my belief that it is too early for me to make a final decision about my own role at Parentline.

PS Evening breaking news: An unpublished paper from SAGE reportedly predicts that, if urgent action is not taken now, there will be as many as 85,000 Covid-19 deaths over the winter months (and in the 'reasonable' worst case projection of Public Health England, 4,000 a day by Christmas) due to the second wave of the pandemic, with the NHS being overwhelmed. Boris Johnson is apparently reconsidering current initiatives in favour of a national lockdown – in new parlance 'circuit breaker'. It remains to be seen how Scotland will figure in all this, but a further total lockdown with 'shielding' seems a real possibility.

1st November

Dramatic announcement last night that the whole of England is going into a 4-week lockdown, precipitating a vigorous debate within the policy community. I wonder how far Covid-19 compliance has become eroded over the last eight months and whether the Tory party may fracture when faced with this new scenario, not to mention the collateral political damage of a destabilising no-deal Brexit!

6th November

The media is absorbed with the protracted indignities of the US Presidential election. As I write, the pundits are projecting a narrow win for Biden, but Trump is threatening multiple lawsuits alleging fraud and seeking to invalidate postal votes that have not already been counted. Meanwhile, amidst similar rancour, England has gone into a second lockdown. It is difficult to see how this can be effective given the continuing inadequacies of the 'test, trace and isolate' system. It is reported that less than one in five of the contacts traced are in fact properly isolating themselves!

Here, in Scotland, we are under Tier 3 restrictions plus additional advice relating to my 'shielded' vulnerabilities. This effectively means we cannot have anyone else in the house or visit others and should not venture outwith the Central Belt.

I managed to join my Parentline Supervisor and a few volunteers on Teams for a catch-up. Their description of the Covid-19 precautions in the shift room was impressive; but somewhat less so when I learnt later in the day that a supervisor and volunteer on a recent shift had tested positive and the permanent team forced to retreat to working from home. It merely reinforces my disinclination to even contemplate returning. My supervisor was not optimistic about my suggestion that I be authorised to do some 'befriending' phone work from home with callers whose main difficulty was loneliness and isolation, subject to the office doing a preliminary risk assessment.

I duly received an appointment for a review of my aortic aneurism. I feel very ambivalent about it. On the one hand, it is potentially lethal if unduly enlarged. On the other, the last place I want to be is in hospital for the scan and certainly for any invasive treatment. It takes all my mental and physical resilience to cope with my Parkinson's Disease.

8th November

Great news. Trump has lost the US election! I hope his humiliation matches that which he has inflicted on so many conscientious members of the US policy community. Biden lacks charisma and youthful vitality but at least he can restore some semblance of dignity and integrity to American leadership. At home, the 'trace and isolate' components of Covid-19 policy continue to miss projected targets. In England especially, there remains a reluctance to use the pre-existing public health and GP network to ensure Covid-19 compliance by contacts, without which the whole lockdown strategy becomes doomed to failure.

Meanwhile, yet another 'horseman of the apocalypse' appears on the horizon! A Covid variant, with no known vaccine, has been identified in both mink and humans in Denmark. The fact that the Danish Government has ordered the cull of all mink in Denmark and that the British Government has immediately introduced additional border controls and quarantine restrictions, says it all.

10th November

An announcement today that a leading drug company [Pfizer] has developed an effective vaccine! Thank God it was only announced after Trump's defeat, although he has yet to concede that he has lost the election and is doing his upmost to rally his supporters to press for recounts and judicial review of the election procedures.

13th November

Yesterday, the number of deaths recorded in Scotland from Covid-19 was at a six-month high and another full lockdown looks possible. Spent the day refereeing an article for the *Journal of Homosexuality* – a desperately inadequate piece with no sense of structure, context or logical continuity. Sadly, I had to recommend its rejection; an option I am always loath to choose as I know from old how depressing rejection can be if you are a young academic trying to get published. But it has never ceased to amaze me how inarticulate research students can be.

Not feeling great these last few days with a lot of muscular aches and pains and feeling stressed. It may be the increased dosage of Ropinirole; hopefully nothing more sinister.

Two slivers of light amidst the gloom; an investigative committee in the USA has found no systemic irregularities in the polling, and Dominic Cummings is ceasing to hold office in Downing Street – a man with a lot to answer for!

17th November

At a personal level, very good news. The scan of my aortic aneurism revealed little change over the last two years and its measurement of 2.9–3.1 would suggest that a 2-yearly monitoring is all that will be required in the future. As the laboratory nurse somewhat drily observed, having established my age, statistically it is almost certain that 'I will die with it, rather than of it'. Meanwhile, I have been occupied completing yet another application to the DVLA. It is unlikely I will do much driving again, but there is something about still being able to if a crisis demanded it that I am reluctant to forego.

Meanwhile, on the Covid-19 front, there is exciting news of more vaccines, although realistically it will be next summer or fall before they can create any significant return to normality. Sadly, there are signs already that they will become the subject of competitive bidding and pharmaceutical warfare, fuelled by the self-seeking rhetoric of populist leaders. The British 'test and trace' process remains an absolute scandal, headed by the inept and beleaguered Baroness Dido Harding. Channel 4 has revealed the continuing failure to exploit the local medical and technical expertise of the established Public Health authorities. Instead, typical of this Government's cronyism, at a cost of 12 billion pounds, the operation has been contracted out to SERCO, who in turn have sub-contracted it to a range of companies that lack clinical experience; including several debt-collectors and Concentrix, a firm whose contract for administering tax credits was previously withdrawn by HMRC. This echoes the earlier breaching of procurement protocols in the purchasing of PPE with contracts worth an estimated 19 billion pounds being arbitrarily allocated to firms associated with Tory party donors and lobbyists.

22nd November

Not a good day for mobility with my feet sticking and feeling very vulnerable. Now up to 18mg with the Ropinirole so some of the problem may be due to side effects.

Trump is still refusing to concede the USA election despite two more states having declared the polls to have been fairly administered! Meanwhile, Johnson is also breaching the normal rules of democratic governance by refusing to sack the Home Secretary, Priti Patel, despite clear evidence that she had created a culture of bullying in several departments of State.

I spent some time this weekend beginning to reflect on my experience as a call-taker in preparation for an interview as part of an external assessment of Parentline. It is good once again to be making a contribution, however small, and to be part of the Whitehouse Loan 'family' once more. It remains to be seen how far the evaluators will appreciate my particular constraints as a call-taker.

We watched a replay of one of the *Plays for Today* from the late 1970s, '*The Black Stuff*'. What a superb film; wonderfully scripted (Alan Bleasdale) and acted (Bernard Hill) and as relevant today as it was then in capturing the fragile and often feral relationships in marginalised areas of the economy and society.

24th November

Again, mixed news about Covid. Deaths from the virus yesterday (608) were at a level only previously experienced in March. But a great breakthrough by the Oxford-Astra-Zeneca Group in developing a new vaccine that might be available for certain groups by the New Year. One can only hope that its distribution will not be as incompetent and prone to cronyism as the handling of PPE and testing!

On the home front, I have been improving my guitar skills and slowly making my way through Hilary Mantel's trilogy on Thomas Cromwell; such a superb piece of writing. I also managed to activate Skype to catch up with M. in Orkney. It was delightful to meet with her online, and a rare opportunity for me to interact visually with someone outwith the home. I used telephone banking for the first time today to wire some money. If this process proves reliable, it will be a godsend as I am increasingly unable to use cheques and my tremor rules out online banking. The Covid guidelines are increasingly confusing and the focus of political criticism, civil discontent and non-compliance. In the last 24 hours Midlothian has suddenly been re-classified as Level 3 with tighter controls imposed with very little notice on hospitality and leisure venues.

1st December

The official start of winter and chaos reigns. In addition to a convoluted set of tiered, so-called 'granular', lockdowns in England, varying somewhat arbitrarily from one local authority to another, Wales, Northern Ireland and Scotland have imposed their own restrictions. In addition, they have all reluctantly agreed to one common set of more relaxed Covid-compliant rules for five days at Christmas! In Scotland, we are now legally forbidden to travel outwith Midlothian except for urgent reasons, ruling out any coastal bird watching that I was contemplating.

The prospect of a no-deal Brexit looms ever larger. It is clear that British firms are not ready to deal with the vast amount of new paperwork that is going to be required. Nor is there any evidence that the Government has recruited the thousands of border officials that will be needed to ensure a smooth transition. There is a real possibility that much of the southern counties will be transformed into one giant lorry park with perishable goods ruined and industrial supply lines fractured. There are also worrying signs that the interests of our fishing and agricultural sectors will be sacrificed in order to obtain some form of trade agreement. Sadly, and ironically, it will be the most ardent Brexiteers, especially in the North of England and in coastal communities, who will lose out most.

Health-wise, my mobility continues to worsen. I am doing more regular exercise on the cycling frame and much enjoying the routine. However, it does inevitably tire my legs and there is a price to pay in weaker synapses later in the day. My tremor overall is marginally improved, but I am still very agitated at the slightest stress and the peculiar agitation triggered by my bowel continues as ever! On the plus side, we were able to obtain a dental appointment at last. Although my teeth clearly could do with some remedial work, the dentist could find no signs of decay or the need for any immediate fillings. As with the nurse at the vascular clinic, the dentist is no doubt working on the principle that my life expectancy does not justify any intervention!

4th December

Suitably apocalyptic start to the day with the first 'Thunder Snowstorm' I have ever experienced.

The first vaccine to be given UK medical clearance (from Pfizer-Biotech) has now arrived! As one newspaper headline put it: 'The needle has landed'. Unsurprisingly, Government spokesmen have indulged in unsavoury attempts to make political capital out of the speed of British validating procedures and even had the temerity to claim that Brexit aided the process. Already, however, it is becoming apparent that rolling vaccination out is far from problem free, not least because there is an acute shortage of clinically trained staff to administer the jag. The Government's priority list is already unravelling as the inability of care homes to cope with an immediate vaccination programme means that the over 80s are likely to be the first group to receive it. One just hopes this is not going to be another little money-maker for Tory cronies. On a more depressing note, well over 600 Covid-19 deaths have been recorded over the last 24 hours and the Chief Medical Officer has warned that the vaccine is unlikely to significantly impact on such mortality rates for another two months, quite apart from the likely resurgence of the pandemic after the Christmas festivities.

The final days of the Brexit transition period are upon us with no sign of a deal. If no deal is concluded, all the evidence suggests that, in the short term, the damage to British industry, finance, and hospitality, and to the standard of living and quality of life, including travel, will be immense, and that there will be a significant shortfall in GNP for years to come, exacerbated by the horrendous deficit incurred during the pandemic.

Spent some of the morning being interviewed about Parentline by a consultancy employed by Children First. It was good to be able to draw on my expertise from over 2,000 hours of call-taking over the years. It made a deal of difference having prepared for the session. In particular, I was able to stress the unique importance of Parentline (highlighted by Covid-19) as a 'first responder' for those requiring emotional support, prior to being signposted to other agencies with legal, financial, and welfare expertise.

9th December

Yesterday, the first vaccine injections commenced in the UK. It remains to be seen how long they secure immunity. I gauge that I fall in the third group to be eligible and that I shall have to wait until next February or March to be inoculated. In the meantime, I need to remain vigilant as the arrival of a vaccine, coupled with the misguided 5-day relaxation of Covid-19 controls at Christmas, will almost certainly encourage irresponsible behaviour leading in the short term to a third wave of infection in the New Year!

I am not feeling good in the mornings. I feel light-headed, faint, and slightly nauseous and my stomach feels tender and bloated. I also have more indigestion and, needless to say, bowel and bladder functions continue to be challenging. In addition, my muscles are aching much more despite the fact that I have temporarily reduced my exercising. Fortunately, as a minor triumph, I managed to secure a phone session with my GP who has arranged for bloods and a urine sample to be tested. It may be the Statins that are causing some of the symptoms, but the most likely culprit is the Ropinirole which I will discuss with my consultant next week in my yearly review; conducted on the telephone.

I feel increasingly neglected by the NHS which, despite official pronouncements, is not 'open for business' for non-Covid patients. This was brought home to me by the news yesterday that one of my oldest friends from my Certificate of Education year (1964–5) at Cambridge, had died in hospital from non-Covid causes without anyone being forewarned of the seriousness of his condition or any proper communication with his wife who was never given the opportunity to talk to him at the end. So, so sad. I woke in the night and was suddenly hit by an awareness of how much I would struggle if anything happened to Mo. It was really the first time that I have acknowledged to myself how dependant I have become. It was only two years ago that I managed to arrange and participate in my book launch. Today, I would not have the physical and social resilience to cope with such an event.

15th December

Across the UK there is now a patchwork quilt of Covid-compliant regulations in so-called 'tiers' varying both across and within regions. London and its environs have now been placed in robust measures, partly due it seems to the impact on infection levels of a new variant of the virus. Along with Edinburgh, Midlothian remains in Tier 3 for the foreseeable future. And yet the Government is still advocating a 5-day reprieve at Christmas in direct contravention of the warnings of its medical advisers that this will merely create a third wave of infection. At the same time, it is clear that Brexit is going to create major disruption in the New Year and panic buying in the supermarkets has already begun. The prospect of a no-deal Brexit combined with ever-changing directives relating to Covid-19 has crucified the leisure and hospitality industries and had a devastating effect on the cultural life of the country.

It is difficult to tease out any positives from the last week. Yet, there have been some upsides. Watching 'The Crown' has been a rewarding experience, not least because I had previously dismissed it as pure 'soap'. Bella has had a few worrying days not eating but seems to have regained her appetite and does not show any distress. She does seem to be sleeping more so we need to keep an eye on her. I would be heart-broken if we lost her! In addition, much to my surprise, the DVLA informed me that they were renewing my license for 3 years! I am entirely unclear as to why they have become more liberal, but it is some consolation to know that I can drive legally if there is a crisis or for some reason Mo cannot be at the wheel. Tomorrow, I am due to have my yearly consultation with Dr Davenport – by telephone. It will be useful to discuss with him my reduced mobility and my decision to reduce my dosage of Ropinirole.

18th December

The call with my consultant was, as usual, brief but focused. Dr Davenport reassured me that, despite various press releases on possible breakthroughs in the treatment of Parkinson's, he did not have any other 'weapons in his armoury' to recommend. He agreed with my current strategy of slowly reducing my Ropinirole until I found an equilibrium between its side effects and benefits. Overall, he felt that I was probably doing better than average. Additional positive news came from my General Practice, with all my tests including cholesterol, prostate, and urine proving normal.

Sadly, the Covid-19 infection rates, especially in the South of England, are rising rapidly, fuelled by the arrival of a new strain of coronavirus (B117), with hospital admittances reaching the peak levels previously experienced in March, prior to the first lockdowns. Recorded deaths from the pandemic now exceed 66,000 with an estimated 200,000 people suffering from the often protracted and life-changing effects of so-called long-Covid. Worryingly, the mutated virus is said to add between 0.4 and 0.9 to the pre-existing R figure, to have as many as 22 mutations and to be 70% more transmissible. The Government's policy on Covid restrictions is a confused muddle. On the one hand they are waiving some of the directives to enable families to meet in their households for 5 days at Christmas. On the other, they are admitting that this will very possibly provoke another wave of infections, leading to the need for yet another nation-wide lockdown in the New Year! Meanwhile, with minimal notice, in England, ill-thought-out schemes for the mass testing of secondary school staff and children in the New Year have been proposed, to be coordinated by the teaching staff. The intention is to employ a 'lateral flow test' that has been widely discredited. Unsurprisingly, this has led to increased confrontation between the teaching unions and the Government.

19th December

London and the South-East of England have suddenly been placed in Tier 4 and locked-down for Christmas. In Scotland, Nicola Sturgeon has reacted immediately to the news that the mutant coronavirus virus has migrated north. The whole of the mainland has been re-designated as Tier 4 and the projected 5-day Christmas relaxation of the rules restricting indoor socialising has been reduced to just Christmas day. From Boxing Day, the whole of mainland Scotland will be effectively locked down for three weeks. Finally, the current restrictions on travel will be enforced throughout the period and from today, with a few exceptions, cross-border travel will be banned! Happy days!

20th December

Some forty countries have now banned any travel from the UK and France has closed off its channel ports. As a result, hundreds of lorries are piling up on the approaches to Dover and Calais. The irony is that emergency plans already formulated for a no-deal Brexit are proving of use. On the other hand, if a deal is not completed in the next few days, without a trade agreement with the EU untold damage to our economy may be inflicted.

24th December

A day of mixed news. There appears to be a Brexit trade deal but there is not good news on the Covid front. Infection levels are rising steeply south of the Border with recorded deaths at unprecedented levels. In addition, a new variant of the Coronavirus, originating in South Africa and with even greater transmissibility, has arrived in the UK.

The day has just flashed by; the usual mix of housekeeping, Skyping, exercising, crossword solving and diary keeping, plus a disastrous game of scrabble accompanied by a very quaffable glass of champagne!

My thoughts go out to the thousands of lorry drivers stuck for days on end near Dover, not to mention the inhabitants of Kent whose roads are in total gridlock and their gardens a latrine for the drivers. It will be interesting to see how far the removal of the recent French border controls in Calais, introduced to prevent the spread of the variant Coronavirus from the UK, will resolve the problem, or whether the final implementation of Brexit will merely prolong the chaos.

29th December

The first snow of the winter, well suited to the chilling news of the pandemic. The new, more contagious strain appears to be spreading exponentially, especially in the South of England. Across the UK, the NHS is struggling to cope, with 5,300 new recorded infections in the last 24 hours. As to the vaccines, they are being developed at an impressive rate but unlikely to impact significantly until the late Spring.

Meanwhile, I have been engaged on the morbid task of putting together a briefing note of my final wishes, including possible speakers and music at the crematorium, and a suggested location for my ashes. With the New Year imminent, there is a growing fear that infection levels will spike again in Scotland, and we must refocus our efforts to stay safe. Sadly, our next-door neighbour has had to go into a care home as she was becoming increasingly distressed and confused. For some time, Mo had shouldered the heavy responsibility of monitoring her but in the end her daughters had to step up to the plate and take control of the situation. As a result, we will now have both houses either side of us up for sale. I pray that the newcomers will be cat lovers! Bella is a wonderful constant in our lives, sharing her affection between us and giving us so much joy. It is hard to believe that we have had her now for 3 years!

30th December

More snow forecast. Again, mixed news of the pandemic. During the last 24 hours, nearly 1,000 Covid-related deaths have been recorded across the UK! At the same time there is encouraging news that the Oxford-based AstraZeneca vaccine has been cleared for use and available for immediate distribution. This may mean some form of protection early in the New Year if adequate staffing for the procedure can be found.

PART II

Variants and Vaccines 2021

2nd January

A surreal start to the New Year as we are very near to being locked down, and human contact is minimal. Mo stood out on the cul-de-sac with neighbours to see in 2021. Sadly, I did not have enough confidence in my balance and tremor to participate. Skype enabled me to keep in contact with Orkney and a Zoom session with my Parentline pals was, as usual, hugely entertaining. I was left, however, with the feeling that I had not been open and honest with them about the possibility that I may well have to retire from Parentline.

The pandemic appears to be overwhelming the NHS down South. Further research has established that the new variant of Covid-19 exceeds the R factor of the existing virus by 0.4 to 0.7, leading to the prospect of exponential growth in the number of recorded cases and deaths, now averaging over 50,000 and 850 per day, respectively. Moreover, the epidemiologists are predicting that the peak may not be reached for some weeks during which we can expect those figures to escalate. The vaccine is, of course, being heralded as the 'game changer', but predictably, as with PPE and 'Test and Trace', there is a lack of coordination and resources to ensure a rapid and systematic roll-out of vaccination, as well as confusion over whether to delay the second injection until the first has been delivered to as many people as possible.

It is very icy on the pavements and it looks as though we are confined to barracks today. Fortunately, I was able to fill the bird feeders yesterday, so it will be interesting to see what birds will be attracted during this cold spell. It would be good to see some redwings and fieldfares.

5th January

We are back to square one! As of midnight, we have been locked down again with legally enforced 'stay at home' orders. Travel is forbidden except when it is a necessity and schools are closed until the beginning of February at the earliest. The only social contact you are allowed is to meet one other person out of doors. Across the UK as a whole the pandemic has been elevated to threat level 5 indicating a real possibility of the NHS being overwhelmed. Compounding the renewed panic surrounding Covid-19 is a concern that the new mutant virus originating in South Africa may not only be more transmissible but also far more resistant to the vaccines now being dispensed. It is all hugely disappointing.

Meanwhile, in the USA, Trump has still not conceded that he lost the election and continues to incite civil disobedience on his behalf. Moreover, a leaked tape records him trying to put pressure on the election officials in Georgia to retrospectively manufacture enough additional votes to support his claim to have won in the State. His behaviour demeans the whole election process in the States and reduces its political ethos to that formerly associated only with unstable third-world countries.

Sadly, one anticipates that Trump's ability to debase the tone of American political discourse is not yet exhausted. He is a sociopathic narcissist and he needs stopping!

On the home front, we finished *The Crown* and are now working our way through *Spiral*. I am just about to register for my 6 months' membership of *Ancestry*, which hopefully will facilitate my efforts to tease out some information on mum.

6th January

Yet another record day for Covid; over 60,000 new recorded infections and over 900 deaths! The total number of recorded deaths from the virus now exceeds 75,000 and, taking into account the overall excess deaths compared with a previous 5-year average, we have, in reality, already exceeded 100,000. The peak will probably not hit Scotland for a few weeks but already it is evident that the NHS is barely coping, with a grim and growing backlog of non-Covid elective treatments. Anecdotal evidence indicates that the police are now adopting a more pro-active and punitive approach to travellers and there is a pervasive feeling of genuine lockdown, especially as the garden in winter cannot provide the same release. [postscript 17.00: Covid deaths for the last 24 hours (of those testing positive within the last 28 days) exceeds 1,000!]

8th January

The perfect storm confronts us. Covid-19 positive tests, hospitalisations and deaths are rising exponentially, and the usual shortfall between promises and delivery is already appearing in the vaccination programme. Similarly, Government assurances with respect to the effects of Brexit on trade and industry are proving illusory. Meanwhile, after the violent invasion of the US Capitol on Wednesday, deliberately incited by Trump in a last-ditch attempt to abort the official recognition of the new administration, one is left with the unnerving knowledge that he is capable of anything in his final days to feed his anger and ego! Some commentators fear he will be tempted to use sympathetic elements of the National Guard to frustrate the inauguration of Biden or make some catastrophic decision to attack Iran. Whatever transpires, his wilful behaviour has let Covid-19 run riot in the States and the Democrats will inherit a volatile and divided nation under relentless siege from the pandemic.

My work on *Ancestry* is proving highly addictive, thanks to the subscription Mo bought me for Christmas. Already I have collected a good deal of information on mum's forbears.

10th January

Again, mixed fortunes. On the one hand, Covid-related mortality levels are increasing every day and now total over 80,000. The rapid escalation in positive tests is now apparent in Scotland, and the mutant virus has clearly migrated north. On the other hand, there is news of the Democrats introducing impeachment proceedings against Trump. Most uplifting though was the sight of a Great Spotted Woodpecker on the feeders and possibly a goldcrest traversing the shrubs at the bottom of the garden!

13th January

Unremitting bad news. There has been a huge escalation in the spread of the new variant Covid. There is acute pressure on ICUs and many thousands of patients on ventilators. Moreover, it is clear that these figures are likely to increase over the coming weeks in spite of the new lockdown regimes. The NHS is in crisis and normal primary care and elective surgery are virtually at a standstill. 50% of the ICU nurses who fought the first wave of the pandemic are experiencing mental health problems, including PTSD. To make matters worse, another mutant Covid virus, thought to have originated in Brazil, has appeared, and yet there are still no stringent immigration controls! It has been calculated that the 'total excess deaths' for 2020, comparing five-yearly averages, is higher than at any time since the Second World War. Further worrying news from the USA where civil insurrection is threatened for Biden's inauguration and Trump continues to refuse to concede defeat or to apologise for his previous inflammatory behaviour. Happily, his erstwhile political and industrial supporters are disappearing like snow off a dyke! It is surreal to see images of the US Capitol akin to those of Iraq after the military invasion with the military stationed on every corner!

16th January

The pandemic crisis deepens with over 47,000 people now being treated in hospital for Covid-related illness. While the peak of infections may have passed, the peak of recorded deaths (now totalling 87,245) is yet to come. ICU departments are struggling to cope and increasingly other aspects of the nation's health are being neglected. The number of patients waiting for elective surgery for over a year has risen exponentially. In response to the worsening situation and in order to defend the UK against the Brazilian strain of Covid, the Government has closed all the existing 'travel corridors' and at long last introduced stringent testing and quarantine requirements on anyone entering the country.

Meanwhile, my days are filled with a wide range of activities; exercising, updating this diary, doing the *Scotsman* crossword, playing the guitar along with Dire Straits, Mudslide Slim, Mark Knoffler and Emilou Harris, watching various episodes on catch-up, and latterly, lengthy investigation into mum's antecedents using my subscription to *Ancestry*.

21st January

Several days of mixed emotions. Huge relief at the departure of Trump and at my invitation to be vaccinated this Saturday. Real concern at the continuing rise in Covid infections, in the number of Covid-related patients in intensive care, and in the associated deaths in the UK, now running at a record average level of over 1,900 per day. In relation to population size, according to some calculations the UK has now suffered a higher mortality rate from the pandemic than any other country in the world. Even with the vaccinations being rolled out, there is little prospect of any real relaxation of the lockdown until after Easter. The danger is that vaccination will delude people into behaving irresponsibly, especially as there is a lack of evidence as to just how long immunity lasts and to what extent asymptomatic sufferers can still convey the virus after vaccination. It is also a sobering thought that, even now, it is estimated that only 17% of those with symptoms of the virus are self-isolating for the prescribed period.

At a personal level the past few days have been dominated by the sudden downturn in Bella's health. We have hopefully now stabilised her respiratory issues with a slow-release antibiotic but there were times when she seemed to have given up the will to live and I was fearful that we might lose her. Mo has shouldered the main stress as she had to take Bella into the vets twice on her own in very wintry conditions and then sit for prolonged periods in the car as the cat clinic has strict Covid-compliant procedures. We would so miss the wee 'torty' if anything should happen to her!

25th January

Not a good 24 hours. Bella was repeatedly sick last night – mainly mucous – and is still not eating. We shall have to contact the vet again tomorrow if she does not pick up. Meanwhile, I am feeling the side effects of the vaccine I received yesterday: aching limbs and general lethargy. The Covid situation goes from bad to worse. There has now been over 100,000 deaths and there are some 40,000 patients seeking treatment in hospital. The number on ventilators is at its highest since the start of the pandemic. The debate surrounding the spacing of the two vaccinations is becoming increasingly fractious, with the BMA criticising the Government's insistence on a 12-week gap for the Oxford Astra-Zeneca vaccine despite the WHO's support for a 3-to-6-week interval.

29th January

Yesterday, we had to make the heart-breaking decision to have Bella put to sleep; so, so, sad. She clearly had some underlying and serious issues with her digestive system and possibly her lungs. Had we kept her, she would, at best, have needed regular medication for the rest of her life and the most likely prospect was that she would suffer a slow loss of weight and the failure of her bodily functions. She was such a delightful, affectionate wee thing; feisty but very beautiful. In all the time we had her (sadly, only 3 years), she never once disturbed us in the night! She was a wee poppet, and we will miss her dreadfully. RIP my little one!

In contrast, there is nothing uplifting in the current confrontation of the EU and UK over the supply of vaccines, nor in the allegations of German medics that the AstraZeneca vaccine is not proven to be effective when given to the over-60s.

A fleeting moment of joy amidst the sadness of this week – a long-tailed tit on the feeders!

3rd February

Missing Bella terribly and still feeling that I let her down and should have argued for one more shot at medication. In my heart of hearts, I know it was the kindest outcome for her, but I grieve for the lovely, spirited girl who brought such joy and was such a companion during my recovery from a stroke in 2018.

The Covid scenario becomes ever-more complex with a variety of vaccines competing for attention. There is an endless debate over their respective efficacies and over the optimal distancing of the two injections. New variant strains are emerging with the increasing danger that the early vaccines will be outmanoeuvred by the virus.

Amidst the gloom yet another moment of sheer delight – the arrival of a goldcrest on our feeders. That flash of gold is pure magic! And for once, it occurred during my participation in the Big Garden Birdwatch!

8th February

The 'beast from the east 2' has arrived with snow and ice and freezing temperatures. The only consolation is that it brings with it a greater variety of birds on the feeders – especially long-tailed tits. My ancestry work continues to absorb great chunks of time, but I am finding details on the female side of mum's ancestry much harder to locate. The Covid situation becomes more complex by the day. Evidence is emerging to suggest that the AstraZeneka vaccine may not provide robust protection against the South African variant strain of the pandemic, and it looks likely that we shall all have to have regular boosters over the next few years to counter the various mutations the virus will inevitably spawn.

Scottish politics is losing its concentration on the pandemic, not least because of the forthcoming Hollyrood election in May. Unwisely, Nicola has now unleashed the IndyRef2 campaigners at a time when her own position is increasingly tenuous given the legal wrangling arising out of the prosecution of Salmond for sexual harassment. Whatever her faults, it is difficult to think of any other Scottish politician who could be as strategic and focussed in handling the pandemic as she has been to date.

11th February

Draconian quarantine measures have now been imposed. All travellers entering Scotland by air have now to isolate themselves in hotel rooms and any evasion of the measures will incur heavy fines and possible imprisonment. Unfortunately, England has only imposed new restrictions on those people travelling from countries on the so-called 'red list', so there is still a loophole through which new Covid variants can spread north of the Border.

We had a substantial fall of snow over the last 48 hours, and it is virtually impossible to take the car out of the cul-de-sac. The situation has been made worse by Morrison's failure to stop and deliver our last order. Mo is apoplectic and hugely stressed. She let them have both barrels over the phone but to no avail.

They failed to call back on several occasions and then cancelled the order without consulting us. I seek solace in the conservatory, birdwatching from my exercise bike. We have begun to watch *Call of Duty* from the very first series – very gripping and a blessed release from Covid documentaries or the impeachment of Trump, and possibly of Sturgeon the way things are playing out!

13th February

Apparently, there is a slight decline in the UK numbers testing positive for Covid, in hospital admittances, and in deaths. However, UK deaths from the pandemic are now well over 116,000 and counting, and the number of patients contracting the disease in hospital is at the highest level since the pandemic began. Today we learnt that in 2020 GDP fell by 10%, the largest downturn since the mini-ice age of the early eighteenth century! In addition, the combination of the pandemic and Brexit is having a devastating effect on firms dependent on the continent both as a market and as a source of components. Problems with the new procedures imposed since our exit from the EU have severely hampered distribution schedules and impacted on the production costs of British enterprises.

Had a lovely Teams session with Gayle and the twins today. It is such a pity that Mo cannot spend more time with them. Last night we were underwhelmed by the take-out from Spoon, and next time we intend to use the Sun Inn. Mo clearly had an adverse reaction from the seafood but fortunately not so severe as to require medical attention. I suspect it is a wake-up call to steer clear of mixed seafood cocktails as take-aways!

19th February

The weather goes from one extreme to the other. The piles of snow that buried the garden last week melted within a couple of days and now we have double-digit temperatures. The Covid situation is complex. Numbers of new infections and deaths are still unacceptably high, but the vaccination programme is making great strides. However, any speedy return to normality can be ruled out, not least because we still do not know for how long these vaccines will convey immunity nor whether asymptomatic patients will still be able to infect others. Nicola is sticking to our semi-lockdown although some children will return to classes next week. The problem is that there is growing evidence that children and young adults are major spreaders of the new variants of Covid, and teachers have not to date been given adequate protection.

My Parkinson's varies worryingly from day to day. Yesterday, my feet were constantly freezing and my hands simply could not play my guitar properly. I assume it is a failure to press the frets cleanly due to a slump in my fine motor skills. What with my dribbling, I feel a decline is upon me. The issue of when and what to say to Parentline is increasingly on my mind. Pushed on with mum's ancestry today and much enjoyed teasing out the details of her maternal great grandfather – a 'hunting and shooting cap maker'.

27th February

Everything is on hold at the moment. We await our second dose of vaccines, but their long-term benefits are still to be defined. Both Boris and Nicola have now introduced new 'road maps' for our exit from lockdown but little has changed in our restrictions.

We are still not allowed to travel more than a few miles and we are still not allowed visitors in the house. It is useless to book anything ahead as there is no guarantee that things will change. If, when the schools go back, the 'I' factor rises again, more lockdowns are inevitable. Meanwhile, with the budget imminent, and with furloughing due to be phased out, the full realisation of the economic cost of the pandemic is about to kick in. It is calculated that we now have a national debt equal to the total value of the economy. The danger is that the economy and markets may crash again. What has yet to be revealed is the full scale of bad debts that will follow from all the loans given out, often without due diligence, over the last year.

The daily melange of ancestry, exercises, guitar, diary, and reading continues. The weather has warmed up and I am hoping to exercise more in the garden. Sadly, and perversely, while using the exercise bike strengthens my legs, it also seems to inhibit the synapses, so I end up freezing more rather than less. I do wonder just what benefit I get from all the Co-careldopa I ingest. I think I might experiment with a slightly lower dose and see what difference, if any, it makes.

The Salmond-Sturgeon Road Show has reached its climax in the Scottish Parliament and it remains to be seen if Nicola will be forced to resign. Whatever the outcome, it is a dangerous distraction when the pandemic is still rampant.

Just spotted that the only engagement I have in the diary for this week is with the podiatrist. How sad is that! Fortunately, my ancestry work keeps me from being bored. I am now entering my third month and still discovering intriguing aspects of my mother's story. This week, rather like a play by Steven Poliakoff, I have been tracking the fortunes of Vernon Harris, my mother's sibling, who disappeared into a mental institution sometime after the Second World War and whose existence was never mentioned in our household thereafter. It appears that in 1951 he was admitted to Lingfield Epileptic Colony in Surrey. As a social historian,

I have naturally digressed to read up on the Colony, originally inspired by Social Darwinist attempts to decant the unemployed 'urban residuum' to more healthy agricultural regimes; then appropriated by neurologists to monitor and rehabilitate patients with learning and other mental disabilities, especially epileptics.

5th March

Having watched the episode of *The Crown* revealing the incarceration of various members of the Bowes-Lyon family with genetic mental disorders to protect the Windsor's reputation, I am even more disposed to find more information on Vernon's hidden existence at Lingfield. Parkinson's a trial today; freezing, dribbling, and poor balance, but managed to keep a sense of purpose; some exercising, some initiating of online chats, some housework, some reading and this update!

Pandemic news is mixed. It appears that most of the vaccines do at least avert hospitalisation in the majority of cases, but yet more variants of the virus are emerging. Meanwhile, the Government is creating mayhem on a number of fronts; precipitating widespread outrage and the threat of strike action by offering the nurses just a 1% pay increase, breaching the terms of the Brexit agreement as it relates to Northern Island, and presenting a budget that completely ignored the crucial issue of social care while pouring public money into investment projects in Tory constituencies won from Labour at the last election – a clear and egregious example of pork barrel politics. The SNP government in Scotland has fared little better with Salmond and Sturgeon locked in combat before various investigations and the party at war with itself. The only upside of this is that the polls are showing a slight fall in the percentage of the Scottish people supporting IndyRef2.

7th March

Started the day progressing my social history analysis of mum's ancestry. It is good to be using my academic skills again. My dribbling is bad and I must remember to avoid sweet things that trigger it off. Weather is not good with high winds predicted. I just hope the pyracantha survives intact.

Covid restrictions are gradually being relaxed but paradoxically those who were formerly 'shielded' are advised to take even more precautions. The medical experts clearly envisage another upswing in cases with the reopening of schools and loosening of visiting restrictions. There is a febrile atmosphere within the policy community and a real danger that the libertarians are going to divert attention from the sober warnings of the CMOs. Meanwhile, we learn today from the Public Accounts Committee that 39 billion pounds! have been invested in a track and trace system in England that is barely fit for purpose and has involved the employment of masses of consultants at exorbitant rates.

'The Harry and Megan Road Show' has been all consuming in the press with public opinion broadly divided. Having recently watched *The Crown*, their complaints seem very credible. I got very upset yesterday when I realised that, along with a significant deterioration in my balance and mobility, my ability to play the guitar clearly had reduced. All I can do is press on regardless as even imperfect fingering will hopefully slow the decline in my fine motor skills.

14th March

Already Brexit is proving a disaster. During the last month exports have declined by 70% and imports by 29%. Our balance of payments deficit is at an historic high and it is estimated that the level of GNP over the last 12 months will have declined by over 9%.

On a more positive note, we have initiated Zoom sessions with my brother and sister-in-law. Its lovely to have visual contact again even if, with both 'aurally challenged', the conversation is a bit of a gong show. This afternoon we watched a superb one-woman performance of *Iphigenia in Splott* online – totally draining but utterly compelling.

18ᵗʰ March

A year ago I started this diary. In many ways not much has changed in our circumstances. For the next few weeks we are still confined to our local area although we can now have a couple round in the garden, if the weather warms up. Big furore has kicked off with many EU countries withholding AstraZeneca vaccines on the basis of false information that it leads to blood clotting, ammunition unfortunately for the anti-vaccine movement. At the same time, supplies of this vaccine in the UK are clearly insufficient to meet the earlier targets of the Government, due to production or perhaps political issues in India. Fortunately, the Government is prioritizing the provision of second doses to the elderly and vulnerable, without which it is likely their immunity would be weak and short-lived.

Today, I drafted my resignation from Parentline and called it a day after 18 years of call-taking. I have found it very upsetting because my weekly shiftwork was hugely satisfying and enjoyable. As with Childline, it was like a family, and I shall never forget the love and affection they afforded me when I had my stroke. My Parkinson's is now compromising my movements so much that I am sure it is the right decision. All very frustrating as mentally I am fine and have no problem with my voice on the phone. Zooming the 'dream team' tonight – I just hope I can keep it together.

Two lovely bonuses yesterday. A family of bullfinches away at the back and visits of a Great Spotted Woodpecker to the feeders!

26th March

I received a delightful response from Parentline to my e-mail of resignation from call taking – wonderfully warm and supportive and with real affection and emotion. My supervisor was equally understanding and sorry to see me go, leaving me feeling I was a genuine loss to the team. So, two emotional hits in one month – the loss of little Bella, my wee joy, and the end of my help-line career. However, good news that I receive my second vaccination tomorrow (who in God's name persuaded the policymakers to use the term 'jab' with all its connotations of an invasive needle!). I am receiving the controversial AstraZeneca version which has become the centre of increasingly fractious exchanges between the EU and UK; no doubt inflamed by the recent hostilities surrounding Brexit.

Nicola Sturgeon survived the recent attempts to bring her down but she has not emerged unscathed and it remains to be seen if the SNP will gain an outright majority in the forthcoming elections. At least the polling seems to suggest that attaining IndyRef2 may not be as straightforward as the SNP hardliners assume.

Nearing completion of my search for mum's ancestry. I have discovered a substantial amount about her forbears and the social history that it reflects, but I am struggling with my personal reflections. The more I try and picture her as a person, the more I realise how little I really knew her. Her contradictions are mystifying. The outgoing confident pre-war bride contrasts with the ever-anxious, self-deprecating post-war wife and mother. The caring, supportive, empathic homemaker was at odds with her many social prejudices encompassing race, class, sex, and disability. She loathed the unions, loyally supported the Tories, and had no time for social 'diversity'. And yet, with her own sons she gave everything. She was always warm and understanding, even when faced with my chequered marital career. She never once put us down and our achievements were always met with pride and endorsement.

27th March

Postscript: Alex Salmond has now created mayhem by establishing a new Scottish Independence Party called ALBA. The knives are really out, and the coming election promises to be a gruesome blood sport! Today, I made excellent progress with the Ancestry manuscript, now embellished with some photos thanks to Mo. I also had my second vaccination that should give me added protection. I cannot help concluding that, with the impending relaxation of Covid restrictions, we are going to import the third wave of infections currently rampant across Europe. So much for sovereignty and taking back control!! At the very least, to combat the inevitable arrival of new variants, we are going to need a series of annual boosters. Deaths from Covid in the UK within 28 days of a positive test now exceed 126,000!

One flicker of normality amongst the gloom – a large sparrow hawk hunting across the garden.

1st April

In many ways the whole saga of the handling of the pandemic might be construed in the future as a one big unbelievable April Fool! Sadly, it is all too real. This week saw the final convincing exposé of the abject failure of 'test and trace' to be fit for purpose despite billions of pounds being expended on it. It appears that less than 20% of those with symptoms of Covid are bothering to take a test and of those testing positive, more than 50% are not bothering to isolate. To make matters worse, a *Panorama* programme this week showed massive contamination of swabs in the testing laboratories with disregard for the integrity of results, under pressure from the Government to focus primarily on ramping up the numbers.

8th April

The AstraZeneca vaccine is fast becoming a political football and entangled with European hostilities generated by Brexit. The medical side effects have been grossly overrated by EU leaders to the detriment of their own vaccination programmes. Meanwhile, continuing lockdown controls, new public order legislation, and the prospect of app.-based vaccine passports being required for entry into public venues have led to growing unrest in the major cities of the country, with violent confrontation with the police. In Northern Ireland, the added frustration over the Brexit protocols and EU trade restrictions are threatening to unravel the Peace Agreement and providing ample opportunities for sectarian thugs to renew their vendettas on the streets.

At home I struggle with my balance and my constant dribbling which adds a new, most unsavoury dimension to my afflictions. Yet I remain positive. I have had three lovely and emotional e-mails from the Parentline team responding to my decision to cease call-taking. They will all be sadly missed. To distract me, I have been making good progress on Mo's father's ancestry, tracking back through the social history of Lancaster in the 19th and 20th centuries. It is amazing how much material one can accumulate from Ancestry coupled with an imaginative use of *google*.

PS: Yesterday, my guitar session went much better. Perhaps it is just that my symptoms vary day by day, but it might also be due to the finger grip exercises I have begun to practise.

11th April

All the media outlets today were dominated by the news of the death of the Duke of Edinburgh leading to a tsunami of overblown, sycophantic eulogies. The usual 'lifetime of service' guff. The only consolation is that, with Covid regulations in place, the funeral will be private and modest. The *Sunday Times* is a depressing read. An excellent article on the SNP and the Scottish economy identifies a series of failed promises and aborted initiatives. Notwithstanding, the SNP is expected by many to triumph in the forthcoming local and Holyrood elections. One can only hope that Salmond's ALBA spoiler party will split the vote!

Feeling under par the last few days and struggling to feel warm. It may be that I am overdoing the Ancestry research and not listening to my body. Sat in the conservatory today reading *Hamnet* for the book group. A good read but too long I think, leading to a loss of momentum at about 70% of the way through. Whilst reading, I had a great sighting of the sparrow hawk hunting across the garden. Meanwhile, my dribbling is a constant irritation as it soaks and marks my trousers. Mo is to have three dental operations on her gums in May. I am hoping that, once she has recovered, we might get another cat, but nothing can really replace my adoring and adorable Bella.

15th April

A lovely day but still a chill wind. As of today, Nicola has decreed that we can travel anywhere in Scotland. My expectation is that all the attractive places to journey to, such as Innerleithen, will be hoatching! It will be great, when the situation has settled, to go to Portobello or Musselburgh, or Longniddry Bents, not to mention old favourites such as Dunkeld or Kirkcudbright.

I received yesterday a wonderful composite farewell card from Parentline – very emotional and affirming. To distract me I am pushing on with the ancestry of Mo's father. It is proving quite challenging as manoeuvring around war records is new to me. But, with the splendid input from Ewan, his grandson, I am making good progress.

The Covid pandemic situation is worrying. The UK figures may be declining but there are new more potent variants appearing from Mexico and India. The latter is a double variant with the potential to outflank our vaccines and it is already in the UK. Most seriously, the new variants appear to be targeting younger age groups. True to form, there is still no ban on Indian travellers coming to the UK! Meanwhile, cronyism knows no bounds within the Tory ranks and the investigation into Cameron's improper lobbying has opened a can of worms; not least the shareholdings of Matt Hancock and his sister in firms granted liberal contracts associated with the pandemic. Clearly our leaders have learnt nothing from the previous debacle over MPs' expenses.

24th April

For the first time since lockdown last year, we went yesterday to Innerleithen, taking advantage of the relaxation of travel restrictions. The weather was ideal and the Innerleithen path ideal for the scooter. Lots of evocative birdsong, especially willow warblers and one chiff chaff. The drive was delightful with very little traffic. Today, we have invited our neighbours to join us for a drink and canapés in the garden. Unfortunately, the weather is not as sunny and warm as predicted. Yesterday was a boost to my physical confidence as I was also able to water the garden without falling! In many ways I am better without a walker as I am more upright and forced to exercise my balance.

The news is dominated by two issues today; Cummings shafting Boris Johnson and the Covid melt-down in India where thousands are dying each day, and the medical services are overwhelmed. Goodness knows what is going to happen when eventually the pandemic really takes a hold in Africa, as it surely will.

27th April

The egregious behaviour of Boris Johnson knows no bounds and he merely hides behind vague and vacuous platitudes about the importance of focusing on the pandemic. In the meantime, our values of integrity and justice are trashed. The whole cabinet is a load of over-promoted cronies with no real commitment to public service beyond their own private ambitions and purses! Meanwhile, the SNP needs to get real. There is no way an independent Scotland could have coped with the pandemic. It certainly could not have funded the furloughing of a significant proportion of the workforce, and with a current deficit estimated at 28% of GNP there is little evidence that an independent Scottish economy would be viable. As one economist commented in the *Sunday Times*, the SNP should drop all the 'virtue signalling' and begin to implement some realistic programmes for recovery.

On Saturday we organised a small drink and canapés occasion in the garden just for the immediate neighbours. This was the first real socialising we had done for over a year. It felt strange not to be too close to others, but it was a very therapeutic experience. I think we are all a little apprehensive about who our new neighbours are going to be either side of us. I just hope they are considerate and cat lovers!

3rd May

Our 24th wedding anniversary. Marked especially by the return of our cleaner; a sign I think of some return to normality. We had friends round for drinks and a take-away meal at the weekend, spaced in the conservatory with some windows open.

My mobility was horrendous yesterday. My feet felt as though they were set in concrete, and it took me forever to get from A to B. It may be that I need to rest more and take naps from time to time. Certainly, my condition varies significantly from day to day. It is the garden and outdoors that I need. In England and Wales, and to a lesser extent in Scotland, restrictions on movement and social contacts are being relaxed in the coming weeks as the level of Covid infections and deaths has fallen dramatically. I fear it may be premature, especially if the Indian variant enters the country. Hopefully, if the situation does not regress, we can enjoy a few days in Kirkcudbright in June, which Mo has booked.

Holyrood and council elections on Thursday. Sadly, the SNP's pitiful economic and social policy record over the last decade will be largely discounted and everything blamed on Brexit and the pandemic. Fuelled by Johnson's repeated duplicity and incompetence and the repellent sight of Tory cronyism, the cause for IndyRef2 will inevitably be strengthened.

7th May

Not a good day for the Labour Party. A disastrous 16% swing in the one by-election, mirrored in the council elections. Keir Starmer clearly does not 'cut through' as the awful vernacular would put it. Meanwhile, there are worrying hints that the particularly virulent Indian (Delta) variant of Coronavirus has established itself in England. The weather is more like winter than spring; barely reaching double figures with occasional thunder and sleet showers. Hence, there is little opportunity to use my scooter. Instead, I have been ploughing on with my research into Mo's father and learning a good deal about the Battleaxe Division and Operation Torch in the process. It appears that at the very same time Ted was participating in the Operation in North Africa, my father was offshore supporting the allied advance in Tunisia until his ship was torpedoed!

8th May

Further dismal electoral news although it does appear that the SNP will not have an outright majority at Holyrood. Salmond appears to have garnered just 2% of the votes and will not gain a seat. Henry Kissinger has a typically insightful commentary on current events when he commented that 'One of the greatest dangers to democracy is the growing gap between those who can win elections and those who can run the state.'

13th May

A mixed day. The Covid news is ambiguous. Boris is pushing his triumphalist line on 'jabs and jobs'; a new mantra that some spin doctor has fed to the front bench. However, a scattering of more sombre warnings from the epidemiologists and virologists about the Indian, so-called Delta, variant does not bode well. The Government needs to act firmly now before it spreads exponentially. Why anyone was allowed into the country from India over the past weeks beggars belief!

My Parkinson's varies from hour to hour, prolonged freezing indoors followed by some fluent walking around the garden. I am considering writing a piece for the *Scotsman* on Parkinson's and the digital revolution that highlights the constraints that those with tremor operate under. A smart phone is now integral to the settling of most invoices but almost impossible to operate with a bad tremor. For the same reason online banking is not an option unless you want to risk adding an extra zero to your payment accidentally. Writing a cheque can also be hazardous. Not only does Parkinson's gradually erode the legibility of your handwriting, cheques as a form of payment are actively disliked by many tradesmen in favour either of cash or a money transfer. Even when I can pay by cheque, my writing is so poor that I am forced to rely on Mo to complete it, other than my signature. The closing of bank branches and ATM points only makes the problem faced by those suffering from a degenerative neurological disease more acute. Even when cash is available, given the pandemic, many traders understandably prefer transactions that are electronic and do not involve the handling of notes and coins.

In contact again with an old school colleague who contacted me out of the blue last year apologising for the verbal bullying he had subjected me to at school. For me, a very conflicted and emotional moment. It brought back the memories of the bullying I suffered over several years that have haunted me all my life. I also felt upset that it was that aspect of the time we spent together that he most vividly recalled. At the time I like to think I showed real resilience and determined to show the name-callers that I would win out in the end, as in one way I did, with promotion to Head Prefect and the award of an Open Exhibition to Cambridge. However, the damage that it did to my self-esteem stayed with me for a lifetime and remains a demon that never fully goes away. It is no doubt this experience that made me so empathic in my handling of bullying calls at Childline and Parentline.

20th May

In the face of the new Indian Covid variant, the Government's much vaunted traffic light system of regulating movement is fast unravelling. The epidemiologists are clearly concerned that the new variant may get out of control despite the extent of vaccination. Meanwhile, thanks to the contradictory messages from various ministers, thousands of holiday makers are heading off to amber-rated destinations and will thereby not only be liable to expensive testing procedures but also a substantial period of quarantine on their return. Good luck to the authorities in policing that!

Two developments on the domestic front. My rather scatter-brained Parkinson's nurse is retiring, and a new nurse has been allocated to me. I am hoping I will get more focused and proactive support from her. Secondly, I have approached Volunteer Midlothian with a view to doing some general befriending calls for them to people in the community who are lonely and isolated. It would be a real boost to my morale to be able to contribute to the community again and use the skill sets I acquired over so many years with Childline and Parentline.

Mo had her first dental surgery on Tuesday. Fortunately, she has recovered well and has confidence in the surgeon doing the work on her gums.

My son is 50 on Saturday! Very sad that I cannot be with him on his 50th; a real marker of how limited the time is that I have left.

29th May

A watershed moment in pandemic politics with Cummings giving his visceral and damning evidence to the Select Committee on the handling of the crisis. Both Johnson and Hancock are singled out for their failure to provide competent leadership and for causing tens of thousands of deaths by delaying the lockdown last year when the medical and scientific advisers had clearly indicated that the pandemic was getting out of control. Cummings was especially virulent in his criticism of Hancock's handling of events, accusing him of repeatedly lying to the Cabinet that the care sector was being protected and that hospital patients were only being discharged to care homes after being tested. The jury is out as to the likely impact of Cumming's evidence on the political situation. Sadly, we are now living in a society where, as in the United States, public opinion has virtually accepted rule by prevarication and vacuous mantras as normal.

On the domestic front, I have had my first (telephone) review with my new Parkinson's nurse who is much more supportive and proactive. She has given me a range of advice to improve the efficacy of my medication. I have also been in contact with Volunteer Midlothian who are keen to use me for befriending calls. I still need to go through the disclosure procedures, but it is very heartening to think that my helpline skillset can still be put to good use.

After a prolonged period of wet and cold weather, this weekend promises to be sunny and warm, and we are looking forward to getting into the garden. Meanwhile, I am nearing completion of my study of Mo's father's ancestry and reading up about the campaigns of the Battleaxe Division of the 78th Regiment during 1942–5 in North Africa, Sicily and Italy, in which he participated. If I can get access to his war memorabilia I could complete the exercise.

30th May

The Government has painted itself into a corner again. Having previously trumpeted the fact that it was following the 'data not the dates', it has now raised expectations of a specific unlocking of restrictions on 21st June. Unfortunately, the Indian Covid variant is spreading fast, and the Cabinet are now faced with another U-turn that will cause a great deal of civil discontent and even unrest, especially in the cities of Northern England. Glasgow also, now effectively the only authority in lockdown in Scotland, may begin to witness escalating levels of civil disobedience.

5th June

An eventful week. Mo had her third dental operation which has left her feeling very sore but hopefully in the long run it will be worth it if she can keep her teeth. The book group met for the first time al fresco, and it was very successful. Almost all the group have ongoing health problems, but the gathering was really relaxed and productive. I found engaging with another pathway and doorsteps was a struggle, no doubt in part due to the impact of the various lockdowns on my physical confidence. I had an informal interview online with the Midlothian Volunteer Coordinator. She is very friendly and affirming and clearly recognises the value of my help-line experience.

My ancestry project continued to progress. I received very interesting material on my uncle's institutionalisation in Banstead Mental Hospital along with details of his diagnosis – 'insane heredity'. I need to do more reading on this to clarify more precisely what it means.

Two disappointing TV experiences this week. The ending of *Line of Duty* was weak and unimaginative, and the first episode of *Ann Boleyn* was flat and unengaging and was far inferior to the TV version of Wolf Hall, let alone the tension and vibrancy evinced by the trilogy of Hilary Mantel.

Postscript: On the pandemic front the traffic light system continues to unravel with Portugal being the latest country to be regraded, with travellers at short notice being required to submit to expensive tests and quarantine on their return. While the level of hospital admissions and deaths has improved, the number of positive sufferers in the central belt has begun to rise sharply, possibly because the Indian variant (now called Delta for political correctness) is more transmissible. There is even talk of a further Nepalese variant that could potentially compromise the vaccination programme. The upshot for us is that Midlothian does not shift down to Level 1 but stays at Level 2 in respect of Covid restrictions.

8th June

Wonderful day yesterday. Taken for an outing to Innerleithen and scootered for over 4 miles. The weather was balmy and Hilary and Martin very attentive. The walkway is superb, and it was so good to get right out of Midlothian. As usual with Hilary, all sorts of goodies appeared, and we picked up the mandatory ice cream en route for home! The day finished with an evening meal at Table Table; the first time since the first lockdown that I have been in a restaurant. Meanwhile, Mo was enjoying some time away. I did not take my binoculars on the walk but saw a group of common terns quartering the river and what I am pretty sure was a northern wheatear with its distinctive while tail. Chaffinches and willow warblers abounded. Back home, the sparrow hawk could be heard 'yikkering' across the gardens. Disappointingly, there appears to be no frogs or toads in the garden pond. I suspect our magnificent grey heron is responsible.

12th June

As I anticipated the prospects of the Government keeping to its much-trumpeted timetable for release from Covid restrictions is fast receding in the face of escalating numbers of those infected with the Delta variant, especially amongst the young. Unbelievably, Dido Harding is putting herself forward to head NHS England!

On the domestic front, Mo's mouth and back continue to cause a worrying amount of pain and discomfort. She has had another scan on her back which hopefully might clarify the source of her condition and is continuing to see her private dentist, in whom she has confidence, albeit at a considerable cost.

A major shift in the sociology of the cul-de-sac is about to happen. Much to our dismay a couple with three dogs have moved in next door with a works van parked in the driveway. At first sight, according to Mo, they seem very nice, but I feel very aggrieved that it puts us in a position where we would be endangering any cat that we might acquire in the future. It is always a lottery, and I must remember that we have had eight peaceful cat-friendly years here. But, with the house the other side of us also available for rental, I think that sadly the chemistry of the neighbourhood will change.

Tomorrow, Gayle and the girls are visiting. It will be delightful to see them again as in a real sense they are our 'grandchildren'. Otherwise, I keep busy and with my freezing bouts the day passes far too quickly. I remain mentally active, with the crossword and scrabble, but also some refereeing; an article for *Scottish Archives* on prostitution in 19th century Aberdeen and a book proposal for OUP on youth sexuality and late twentieth-century family planning provisions. Needless to say, the remuneration is minimal but the value for me lies in keeping in touch with new scholarship in the history of sexuality.

15th June

Yet again, you could not make it up. Having nominated a day for the 'irreversible relaxation of Coronavirus' restrictions Boris has now had to backtrack in the face of the Delta variant and suspend the process for an additional month! 19th July, my birthday, is now designated the 'Terminus' for all Covid restrictions. We shall see. In Scotland, Nicola has likewise deferred the anticipated freeing of controls scheduled for 29th June for a further three weeks. Meanwhile, that vacuous excuse of an international trade minister, Liz Truss, has become positively orgasmic over her so-called free trade agreement with Australia; an agreement that will possibly undermine the viability of UK farmers and is calculated to add to our National Income by a staggering 0.02%!

24th June

A sense of calm before the storm. Although the Cabinet are hell-bent on keeping to their much-vamped 'Freedom Day', the level of infections is rising ominously in Scotland. In addition, there is evidence of a new vaccine-avoiding Covid variant – labelled the Delta plus variant – that is reported to have emerged from Nepal. To add to our woes, the medical experts calculate that there are now two million people in England suffering from long Covid, who represent a huge challenge in the coming months to the NHS on top of the anticipated return of winter flu. Meanwhile, Boris continues to undervalue the seriousness of the situation and relies on populist soundbites to deflect criticism. His latest mantra, no doubt dreamt up by some waster in the Cabinet Office, is that 'The Government jabs while the Labour opposition jabbers'!

25th June

It transpires that the number of new infections over the last week in the UK is at unprecedented levels, albeit the number of hospitalisations and deaths is being constrained by vaccination. Indeed, the UK level of virus spread is higher than any other country in Europe. To add further irony to the Covid saga, it appears that Hancock has been having an illicit affair and indulged in some frottage that he has condemned in others! Unsurprisingly, Johnson has supported him but the credibility of

Hancock's position as a health minister preaching self-control and distancing may have been fatally damaged.

We are about to go to Kirkcudbright for a few days; the first proper venture out in eighteen months. It will be lovely to see some of our old haunts again but also a challenge given the deterioration in my balance and mobility and my increasingly unsavoury habit of dribbling.

4th July

We had a lovely 3 days in Kirkcudbright: challenging but rewarding. Our moods were both enhanced by having some time away together for the first time in 15 months. The self-catering apartment was far from perfect, but it was perfectly located across the road from the Selkirk Arms. The weather for once was brilliant and we spent one idyllic afternoon by the river, albeit only after we had to negotiate curbs that were not designed for mobility scooters. For some reason the town was incredibly busy on the Monday, which behove us to be constantly vigilant about sanitising, masking and distancing.

Regarding the pandemic, I fail to comprehend what the Government's policy seeks to deliver. At a time when the number of infections is rising exponentially, and with low compliance with a 'test and trace' system that is not fit for purpose, they are continuing to present the 19th of July as 'Freedom Day', when most restrictions will be lifted. They argue that by then a major proportion of the population will have been vaccinated and therefore new infections will not, as before, lead inexorably to increased hospitalisations and deaths. However, it is far from clear that the current vaccines will cope with new variants of the Coronavirus. Moreover, with NHS staff already exhausted and under-resourced and routine elective surgery now subject to unprecedented delay, even a modest increase in hospital admissions is likely to overwhelm the Service. Nicola Sturgeon is reluctant to be bulldozed into complying with the English timetable for exiting restrictions, not least because the daily increase in the number of those infected in Scotland, (as of yesterday, c. 4000), is now the highest since the start of the pandemic. What is worrying is that, politically, the temptation is to opt for the relaxation of restrictions notwithstanding the views of medical experts, partly to placate an increasingly vocal group in society who threaten to indulge in civil disobedience if their freedom of movement is not restored.

The appropriately named Hancock has been forced to resign; ironically for not adhering to his own diktats on 'distancing'. Meanwhile, Gove is seeking a divorce from his journalist wife, Sarah Vine, who aptly reflected on the 'aphrodisiac of power' in a recent article. It was ever thus!

6th July

So, we now have a new mantra: 'Learning to Live with the Virus'! The Cabinet has done a complete U-turn and prioritized date over data, announcing, contrary to much expert advice, that from 19th July there will be an 'irreversible' lifting of Covid restrictions in England including social distancing and the wearing of masks. The onus of responsibility to avoid the spread of infection will now rest with the individual citizen rather than official directives. This, despite a 70% rise in infections in the last week. In Scotland, Nicola has set her next deadline somewhat later in mid-August. However, the WHO has now listed Scotland as one of the worst epicentres of the disease, in large part attributable to Scottish football fans attending the Scotland-England match in Wembley, and it is difficult to see how the First Minister can possibly stay in line with the wild and premature announcements south of the Border.

9th July

The Government has now taken the huge gamble of promising to remove lockdown restrictions in England after the 19th of July and to loosen the operation of self-isolation. The wearing of face masks is also to be left to individual risk assessment and not the law. And all this at a time when the level of new infections is spiralling with the R rate calculated to be between 1.2 and 1.5. Moreover, there appears to be a reversion to some sinister form of eugenic/herd immunity approach to the new mantra of 'living with the virus'. Unbelievably, Cabinet Ministers are assuming that infection rates may rise to a daily increase of 100,000 a day by August. They are relying on the hope that the connection between infection and hospitalisation will continue to be broken by vaccination. Already there is a strong backlash from the Labour leadership, from many Trade Unions, from the Metro Mayors, and from NHS managers and medical experts, not to mention the Covid bereaved. There is real concern that those suffering from auto-immune conditions will have to 'shield' once again; that allowing such large levels of infection to circulate unchecked will encourage the emergence of new more resistant variants, and that the increased demands on the NHS will further delay elective surgery, the backlog for which is now estimated to involve over 5 million cases!

In Scotland, several hospitals have already issued a Code Black. There is also the possibility that new variants will target younger age groups who have not yet been vaccinated, and at best leave many youngsters with long-term medical issues. At the moment another key issue is that, with a sudden rise in the number of positive cases that will follow inevitably from the relaxation of pandemic restrictions, increasing numbers of health workers and other key workers will find themselves 'apped' and have to self-isolate. Predictably, the Government's solution to this problem is to order that the sensitivity of the test and trace application be weakened, thus compromising the whole purpose of the process.

My balance has been especially bad this week along with my freezing. Sometimes, I can barely move, and any task is hugely time-consuming. I am befriending another Parkinson's sufferer as of next week and it will be good to compare notes on how we are faring – it promises to be a real 'organ recital'! To add insult to injury I have had to struggle online with my application for a new Blue Badge that I foolishly forgot to apply for well in advance. You would think, knowing the type of person applying, they would make the form simple, but far from it. Even the formatting of the form was a nightmare, and I can only hope that my soft-soaping of the support officer who was processing my application pays off! [Postscript: It did, and my badge was issued within 24 hours thanks to my having identified a support worker with whom I could liaise].

16th July

A very mixed week. The preparation for 'Freedom Day' has led to a fracturing of much of the consensus that prevailed after the first and second lockdowns. Much of the modelling on which Johnson's reckless removal of restrictions is based assumes catastrophic levels of infection that can only be contained by vaccination, and we have no certain knowledge that another more resistant strain of Coronavirus is not going to emerge. Over the last week the level of new, recorded infections in the UK has risen by 70%. Many of the medical experts have stressed that, along with a predicted rise in flu and respiratory diseases by the autumn, the pandemic is liable to overwhelm a health service that was already at full stretch and desperately under-resourced when Covid-19 appeared on the scene.

My own health is increasingly compromised by Parkinson's. As I said in my application for a Blue Badge, I 'totter' rather than walk and I am increasingly subject to 'freezing' for seconds, and frequently minutes, at a time. My dribbling has also become a real issue. Once I have come off Ropinirole entirely I intend to seek advice from the Parkinson's nurse to see if she can suggest some alternative medications.

But all has been put into perspective by the serious illness of our granddaughter in Canada. She has had a burst appendix' and the level of associated infection is such that they cannot yet operate on her. She is critically ill, and we fear for her and for the trauma they are all going through.

My new role as 'community connector' is taking time to progress. So far, no suitable match has been found for me.

The ancestry work proceeds apace. I have now mapped out the story of three generations of Amy's paternal ancestry but I think the maternal side may prove to be a much more difficult task. However, I have learnt a great deal about rural Perthshire in the process and we plan at some point to drive around to see all the farmsteads and bothies where Mo's forbears toiled for a living on the land, a total contrast to the London and Lancaster-based histories of my previous efforts.

26th July

Really struggling today. I had a bad night with the frequent need to pee and, coupled with my increasing difficulty in getting out of bed, I was exhausted and very faint when I first got up. Fortunately, after an extra hour in bed and some breakfast I feel better, but I must talk to the Parkinson's nurse and see if there is any other medication I can try. I am also having real problems negotiating the slight step in the garden. It is all in the mind but crippling for all that.

A new word to add to our Covid lexicon: 'pingdemic'. It has arisen out of the risible handling of 'test and trace' in England. Predictably, as the number of new infections has been allowed to rise, so has the number of workers forced to isolate due to being contacted on their 'apps' irrespective of whether they themselves have had both vaccinations and tested negative. As a result, many key sectors, especially distribution, are suffering acute shortages of staff and this is impacting on the availability of food and other necessities. On top of the byzantine regulations now imposed by the EU on British exports, this has led to a perfect storm for British industrial and commercial enterprises.

Good news from Canada. Ella is home and her appendix will be removed within sixty days when her infection has been completely eradicated. Such heartening news trumps all my whingeing!

4th August

The Parkinson's is leaving me low and agitated with dribbling a constant irritation and reminder of how very slowly my bodily functions are shutting down. Even making this entry is a challenge.

The process of relaxing travel and distancing restrictions is ongoing, but I have little confidence that it is truly informed 'by the science'. I suspect it is largely a function of political opportunism and it would never surprise me if Boris suddenly decided that he had enjoyed sitting in the Prime Minister's seat, thank you very much, but now it was time to reap the financial fruits of office and to retire to the lucrative world of public speaking and board membership. However, I think his cronies will want to keep him in his post long enough to soak up the responsibility for the broken promises of Brexit and the parlous handling of the pandemic.

It was lovely to see Gayle and the twins at the weekend. Mo was wonderful with the children and Gayle is so caring and appreciative. I hope, if Mo can gain confidence as to the route, that she might be able to look after the girls one day a week. I would have to be very organised to ensure my safety.

Sadly, the cul-de-sac has lost some of its appeal. Our new neighbours have three dogs and run a roofing business from home, monopolising parking space. They regularly smoke cannabis, and their behaviour leaves a lot to be desired. During our absence the other week, they apparently introduced a dose of Eastenders to the cul-de-sac with a shouting match at midnight in the street culminating in those immortal words: 'You are nothing but a f...ing whore!!' Such are the narrow confines of our present lives that the major issue now being addressed on WhatsApp is whether they should be invited to the communal barbecue. How sad is that?

9th August

Torrential rain yesterday on our journey to Comrie but it was a relief to see Perthshire again. I managed to survive the trip without incident and found that, outwith the house, I can avoid freezing. I think it must be that in open spaces I have momentum, but it is also about how focused my mind is. At home, I am always thinking ahead about what I need to do and what next I need to explore on *Ancestry*, and this cuts the synapses.

Hilary's birthday today. I cannot believe that she is 47! A belated Zoom with Canada last night. Ella still looks very pale but thankfully is out of danger. Meanwhile, sad news of my old mate, Tony, who has just had a stroke. I will ring him later, but I gather his stroke was a mild one.

Scotland's so-called 'Freedom Day' today with the removal of Covid restrictions but I sense that Nicola is still very uncertain about the ability of the health service to cope with another rise in the number of people testing positive which is anticipated with the new freedom of movement, the end of distancing, and the reopening of the schools. The prospect of a virulent flu epidemic this coming winter is an additional concern.

16th August

A week graced by more socialising with old colleagues and long-standing friends from Edinburgh University. It was delightful to catch up with news from the department, which predictably no longer exists as a separate entity. I am just grateful that I retired when I did as the unit of resource has steadily deteriorated and the demands on lecturers are hugely more exacting; quite apart from the increased workload associated with the pandemic and online teaching. We have sadly lost the collegial atmosphere that we once enjoyed in our respective Faculties.

However, the pandemic has had its cultural advantages, not least in the development of online access to book festivals. Yesterday, we signed into two excellent presentations in the Edinburgh Book Festival – Joan Bakewell (in less politically correct times, widely regarded as 'the thinking man's crumpet!') on planning for the end of life, and Tom Devine on Scottish historiography. Over the next two weeks we have registered for a range of sessions that enable me to enjoy the festival without the stress of having to travel into Edinburgh, and associated bladder issues.

I have slowed the pace of my ancestry work and feel the better for it, as does Mo. It has enabled me to take stock and focus more effectively on the crucial gaps in the narrative.

In particular, I would dearly like to consult the documents left by Ted relating to his active service in the Battleaxe Division in World War 2.

A sad, sad day for Afghanistan and one that Biden could ill-afford, even if the decision to withdraw was initially that of Trump. Echoes of Vietnam and the flight from Saigon!

20th August

Some worrying straws in the wind. The Greens have done a deal with the SNP. In return for a share in government, they will ensure that the SNP has a working majority at Holyrood, thus enabling an early attempt to force through IndyRef 2. This, at a time when the Scottish economy is running a 37-billion-pound deficit equivalent to 24% of GNP. But as Tom Devine recently observed, the experience of Brexit demonstrated that populist fervour can these days readily trump harsh economic reality in shaping public opinion.

21st August

Two delightful experiences today: a mob of long-tailed tits on the feeder, and a superb performance by the National Theatre called *Hansard*. The play, set in 1988 at the time of the Local Government Bill outlawing the mention of homosexuality in school sex education, combined some of the funniest satire and visceral personal exchanges – a truly memorable production.

24th August

Off to Innerleithen today for a scoot. The weather looks fine and promises to be hot. Despite my balance issues I managed to load the scooter by myself which is good for my confidence, but I am feeling quite light-headed. We held the cul-de-sac barbeque on Sunday despite the rain. Everyone was very supportive. Our new neighbour made an effort to introduce himself (somewhat inappropriately by shaking my hand!!) but he looked uncomfortable, and I have my doubts as to how far his family will integrate into the community. I sense that the feel and sociology of the cul-de-sac will change.

My volunteer role as Community Connector still has not started and the coordinator seems to be constantly struggling to obtain a match for me. However, there is no urgency and I have plenty of other supportive calls I should make. The apple-coring season has started early this year, and this is thankfully one task I can perform. There looks to be many hundred weights of apples on the tree, so I am going to be kept busy for several weeks.

25th August

The outing to Innerleithen was hugely enjoyable. As always, the drive there was beautiful, with the purple heather set against the green hills. Saw a flock of linnets and two ravens and what may well have been a redstart.

Two sobering developments on the Covid front. Yesterday saw the highest recorded new cases in Scotland since the pandemic began. In addition, it appears that the protection afforded by the vaccines only lasts a few months and it is likely that we shall all need a booster in the autumn. Worryingly, nearly half of new infections now involve people under the age of 25. Significantly, our podiatrist requested we put masks on yesterday for her visit; the first time for some months.

30th August

A bitty day largely due to my lack of balance and the inordinate time it takes me to get from A to B. Spent some time with Mo listening to some episodes of the podcast on the Nuremberg trials. Odd to recall my first sight of Nuremberg some years ago on our Viking cruise. What struck me most was how completely the Germans had been able to reconstruct their city in comparison with the dilatory rebuilding of many of our urban areas. 'To the victors the spoils' was an aphorism that did not seem to apply.

As I anticipated, the number of new Covid cases in Scotland is rising rapidly – yesterday exceeding 7,000! Already, normal primary care and elective surgery is again being impacted. Scottish towns and cities now occupy six out of ten of the leading sources of infection in Europe. However, we are now facing increasing and widespread resistance to any further lockdowns and a growing belief in many areas of the policy community that we may just have to live (and die) with the virus if we are ever to restore the economy and the fabric of civil society. As the headline in the Scotsman summed up the situation, we are faced with a 'Perfect Storm'.

2nd September

There are already signs that the pandemic is threatening once again to overwhelm the health services. In the UK recorded deaths due to the virus are again running in excess of one thousand a week and Scotland continues to figure prominently in the list of European viral hotspots. Yesterday, Nicola Sturgeon announced that in Scotland vaccine passports would be needed for entry to nightclubs and large gatherings from the end of the month. I suspect that this is but the start of a retreat into another damaging and contentious lockdown.

Meanwhile, the weather continues to be dry, with very warm sunny periods especially towards the end of the day.

4th September

I am conscious of the nights drawing in and the prospect of another winter. My walking is now declining fast and barely more than a totter. I feel increasingly vulnerable to contracting the virus because of the relaxation of restrictions and the increase in informal gatherings. Two members of our book group, with whom we have socialised in the last 10 days are unwell; one of whom has tested positive. What the outcome will be in terms of our needing to isolate, remains to be seen. I pray that we don't get infected.

The political scene is becoming increasingly confused and febrile. Government spending in 2020–21 was at an historic high of 54% of GDP and the Government is now split over whether, contrary to their manifesto pledges, increases in national insurance and a suspension of the triple-lock on State pensions are needed; especially given the need to gain some traction on the contentious issue of the funding of social care. Another area of contention is the question of how far vaccination should be extended to teenagers; this at a time when distribution problems are already threatening to delay the rollout of annual flu vaccinations. I have decided to cut down on listening to the news and instead to sit and listen to classical music.

9th September

Watching footage of the 9/11attack on the Twin Towers is still a surreal experience. Sadly, with the recent retreat from Afghanistan it is evident that little has been learnt from the experience. Still more depressing is that the community solidarity that marked the aftermath of 9/11 has been fractured by Trump and the USA left a divided and rancorous nation.

Today, it was announced that Scotland has now an unprecedented level of Covid infection and that one in forty-five people in Scotland are currently suffering from the pandemic. I seriously doubt whether Nicola can let its incidence further escalate without imposing another round of controls. Given the scale of the problem, the introduction of vaccine passports, made possible, be it noted, with the two-faced, opportunistic support of the Greens, will prove to be a fruitless exercise.

12th September

I was privileged last night to watch an awe-inspiring performance by Emma Raducanu in the United States tennis open championship, a truly historic display of power, positioning and poise.

Today, very worrying news from Canada. Ella still has some infection and can suffer an acute appendicitis at any time. She is scheduled to have her appendix out in October. In addition, they have detected an anomaly in her stomach that was not there on previous ultrasounds. The medics do not think it is serious and most probably a benign cyst that they will remove along with the appendix. Nonetheless, I can only imagine the stress and upset the family must be going through.

For the first time in a long while I saw a greenfinch on the feeders today.

15th September

Liz "*I know*" Truss as Foreign Secretary!! The world has gone mad!!

16th September

NHS in Scotland not looking good. The average time for an ambulance to come is now over 6 hours and Nicola is considering calling in the military to help out. England has begun to introduce booster vaccinations and I hope Scotland will follow suit without delay.

27th September

Autumn is well and truly on us, and the apple tree is heavily loaded. Just back from spending a few days in Kirkcudbright. A mixed experience. My movements were pitiful and can most appropriately be characterised as festination, freezing, and f... ked! We also wasted a day while the heating was fixed. On the plus side we had a very enjoyable time hosting some close friends. Hilary and Martin also came to stay a couple of nights and were great company. Unfortunately, Mo had to do more cooking than was planned as all the restaurants were booked out; no doubt a function of 'staycation'. We did manage to get to the RSPB Mersehead reserve and use the scooter but due to the recent absence of rainfall there was a lack of wetland and consequently few geese.

Meanwhile, there is a new panic relating to the shortage of petrol and diesel with filling stations running dry due to distribution problems brought on primarily by Brexit. As a result, the Government has been forced to deploy army personnel as drivers and to issue emergency visas to enable continental drivers to operate once again in the UK. It is a humiliating mess. The Labour Party Conference threatens also to descend into chaos with Keir Starmer's deputy behaving like a fishwife and Jeremy Corbyn's rabid, anti-vaccine brother gate-crashing proceedings. Starmer's reasoned, forensic style, reminiscent of the Fabian Society of old, fails to 'cut through' as the modern parlance would put it. Although he has successfully altered the rules relating to the leadership selection within the Party, he has still to win the confidence of the rank and file of the Movement and remains way behind Boris in the popularity polls.

1st October

Autumn gales have arrived along with kilos of fallen apples that Mo is distributing around the cul-de-sac. I have now completed my third ancestry study – of Mo's mother. In many ways it has proved the most challenging as generations of agricultural labourers left little footprint in the records, but along the way I have learnt a great deal about the social history of rural Perthshire in the 19th and early 20th centuries.

It is a challenge to be positive about current affairs. A combination of Brexit and the pandemic has produced acute supply problems, both in terms of labour and materials, across many sectors of the economy; the most recent being shortages of petrol and diesel on the forecourts, of building materials in the construction industry, and of butchers and abattoir workers for meat processing. My best guess is that all these supply constraints, coupled with the global hike in gas prices, will lead to inflationary pressures and a rise in the cost of living and interest rates. In turn, this will impact on the many borrowers who have previously enjoyed low interest rates and inevitably lead to foreclosures and bankruptcies and another financial crisis. This may well be exacerbated by the collateral damage from an anticipated collapse in the Chinese property market. As Mo would say: 'Ever the optimist'!

4th October

The Tory annual conference has produced a whole new spate of vacuous mantras including 'levelling up', 'building back better', and 'getting on with the job'! The reality is that Brexit has created a ruinous scenario for many firms and the Tories' declared aim of a low tax, controlled immigration, high wage, high skilled, high productivity economy is a pipedream. The fact that inward investment in the UK economy is running at only 0.1% of GNP says it all.

At a low ebb yesterday. My mobility and balance were so poor that for the first time I talked to Mo about the need to consider purchasing a wheelchair for indoor use. On a more positive note, my telephone befriending went well, and it felt good to be exercising my helpline skills again.

11th October

Autumn has now set in with a vengeance with a constant fall of apples on the lawn. Telephone befriending went well again today but I need to arm myself with more chat lines as Do has, faute de mieux, little activity from one week to another. Tomorrow,

I introduce Damian Barr's *Maggie and Me* to the book group; meeting face to face for the first time since March 2020! I only hope my tremor does not kick off. It is an inspiring book in many ways and poses the question as to how some people from abusive backgrounds have the resilience to survive and flourish. I do think though his identification with Thatcher's call for individualism and sheer determination as opposed to systemic social change is misplaced. There *is* such a thing as society and to identify with her ruthless free-market libertarianism as inspiring is to do his story an injustice.

The Government continues to stumble from one crisis to another. The latest threat is from the dramatic escalation in wholesale gas prices due to acute supply constraints, with the consequent erosion of profit margins across industry, together with the collapse of energy firms restricted by a statutory price-cap and the prospect of rapidly spreading fuel poverty. Predictably, Boris has chosen this time to go on holiday while the Treasury and Business Secretary are at each other's throats over how far the State should intervene with yet another round of financial support. Add to this our alienation of the French and EU over trade negotiations, and our threat to renege on our commitment to the Northern Ireland Brexit Protocol, and you have a thoroughly beleaguered nation. And yet Boris still leads by a mile in the polls!

12th October

The total deaths in the UK attributed to the pandemic have now reached in the region of 140,000. More significantly, the newly published report of two parliamentary select committees concludes that the handling of Covid-19, and especially the delay in introducing lockdown in 2020 and the subsequent inadequacies of 'test and trace', constituted the UK's 'worst ever public health failure'.

17th October

A productive few days. I have enjoyed indulging in more reading, both popular and academic. Unfortunately, the more thought-provoking the read, the more my movements freeze! I am also gaining huge solace from observing the bird feeders. In addition, I have decided to read slowly through my volumes of the *Journal of the History of Sexuality.* It is a luxury after all these years not to have to take notes.

Two engagements have been announced. Much to our delight, my lovely goddaughter, Susie, has become engaged. Coincidentally, my grandson, has proposed to his girlfriend. We have barely seen him over the years but wish them every happiness.

21st October

The leading medical agencies, including the BMA, are putting increasing pressure on the Government to reintroduce Coronavirus restrictions in England. The number of people testing positive is spiralling again and approaching 50,000 cases a day. Even though the level of hospitalisations and deaths has not reached the peak of last March, it is clear that, with the onset of flu cases and the need to catch up on the huge backlog in elective surgery and GP consultations, the NHS is in crisis. The Government is trying to brave it out for fear of losing face, and despite anticipating 100,000 new cases a day in a few weeks' time, they are refusing to implement 'Plan B' which would again require the compulsory wearing of face masks, proper distancing, and proof of vaccination for larger venues. They continue to assert that the situation in the NHS is 'sustainable' while the death toll mounts. An added concern is the emergence of yet another variant, AY.42, that is more transmissible than the Delta variant. Personally, I shall be glad to have news of the booster vaccinations given that there is increasing evidence that the immunity conferred by our initial injections, especially those using the AstraZeneca vaccine, will soon disappear.

27th October

A great deal has happened since my last entry. The Westminster Government has resolutely refused to reintroduce restrictions despite ever-growing advice to the contrary. In Scotland many of the restrictions still apply but there appears to be widespread disregard for the need to wear masks especially on the trains. Meanwhile, the COP26 Climate Change Summit is due to start in Glasgow even though it will almost certainly prove the epicentre of a new outbreak of the virus, and indeed possibly a new variant given that thousands of people will be flying in from all around the world! Given that Glasgow cannot accommodate a significant proportion of the delegates, it is likely that Edinburgh will also see a spike in the incidence of the virus. This, at a time when the Scottish Health Boards are lobbying Sturgeon to enlist the army for support as they are operating at full capacity. Not before time a Commons Select Committee has vilified the 'Test and Trace' operation that cost 37 billion pounds with no discernible effect on the spread of the pandemic, thus necessitating the lockdowns. The use of private consultants at extortionate fees merits more forensic investigation as the whole operation smacks of cronyism and corruption; all at the taxpayer's expense.

We have now had our boosters with no side effects. As of next week, our immunity should be at about the 90% level. Sadly, my balance and freezing has again deteriorated, and I have had two falls in the last 10 days. We are off to Crieff Hydro tomorrow and I am very concerned as to how I will cope at mealtimes. The falls have severely undermined my confidence.

1st November

The stay at Crieff with Gayle and the twins was delightful despite the atrocious weather. It was lovely to play the loving grandparents for a few days and to have some quality time with them. Ava and Cara are real characters and clearly very relaxed with us. We used the scooter indoors for the first time to great effect. The staff were hugely supportive and facilitated my access whenever it was needed. I am really struggling now to achieve any fluidity of movement and maybe the time has come to explore the possibility of acquiring a small slim wheelchair for use indoors.

5th November

Yesterday, I returned at last to Vane Farm courtesy of Paul's wonderful support. I managed to take the scooter into all the hides. The weather was excellent; cold but a clear bright light for bird watching. The usual suspects: teal, widgeon, mallard, tufted duck, pochard, golden eye, and great crested grebe, but no pintail. Great view of whooper swans and the day's special, a marsh harrier quartering the reeds in front of us. The main challenge of the day was my bladder and the difficulty of having sufficient layers of clothing to keep warm while gaining easy 'access' for a pee!

The main news today was the abject failure of Johnson to protect an ex-minister from sanctions imposed by the all-party Parliamentary Standards Committee in view of his lobbying activities. The whole episode has 'sleaze' writ large and there are murmurings in the Tory backbenchers that the party leadership may be losing credibility.

8th November

The Westminster outcry against Johnson's casual disregard for the reputation of Parliament is likely to find voice today when the issue of disciplining members' behaviour has been accorded a separate debate. Of especial interest will be the call for an investigation into the Covid-related contracts awarded to the firms for which Owen Paterson was lobbying.

Meanwhile, there is a growing disjuncture between the Government's grandiose claims with respect to social levelling and betterment and the economic facts. The Resolution Foundation has found that, in the period of the 2019–24 Parliament, growth in real household incomes will grow at a mere 0.1% a year; the weakest performance since the data became available in 1955. As a leading Scottish economist has observed: 'This is as close to stagnation as you can get'.

15th November

The days are fast drawing in and winter beckons. I will miss the hours spent in the conservatory but hopefully I may get to Vane Farm once a month. On the Covid front, there are mixed messages. The politicians stick to a cautionary stance but deny any imminent prospect of another lockdown, relying on the vaccination programme to keep the situation under control. In contrast, NHS managers argue that the service is at crisis point and unsustainable at current levels of demand. A further wave of the pandemic is sweeping westward across the continent with new lockdowns in countries such as the Netherlands and Austria and it seems highly likely that it will wash up on our shores. People with strokes and heart attacks in the UK are having to wait on average over 50 minutes for an ambulance and then a further wait, sometimes of many hours, before they are admitted to A&E. Waiting times for elective surgery such as hip replacements are now predicted to be as long as five years. Meanwhile, the care sector is critically short of staff; a situation only exacerbated by the Government's insistence that all care workers must be vaccinated.

The sleaze debacle continues apace and appears to have 'cut through' to the electorate, with the most recent polls showing Labour inching ahead of the Tories. Some of the economic performance figures belie the picture painted by Tory spokesmen. GDP rose by only 1.3% in the third quarter and it is estimated that the economy has declined by over 5% compared with pre-pandemic times. Another worrying development is the rise in the inflation level to nearly 5%, about double the Bank of England's target. This will inevitably lead to a rise in interest rates at some point, confronting thousands of homeowners and small businesses who have borrowed in a period of historically low rates with imminent bankruptcy. One ray of sunshine amongst the gloom; it appears that there is still no clear majority in favour of Scottish independence.

My condition continues to vary from day to day. I am trying to use a cane rather than a walker as much as possible as it is better for my posture. I have been trying to collect some Christmas presents for Mo and making good progress. However, it is evident that for some purchases (for example, concert bookings) you need to have a smart phone to process e-tickets using an app. that I do not have. It is only a matter of time before I will be as 'disenfranchised' as those who have no access to a computer!

21st November

A fresh wave of the pandemic is now sweeping across Europe with a range of new restrictions and lockdowns being introduced in many countries. These are being violently opposed in Austria, Germany, and the Netherlands. The WHO has warned that unless controls are reintroduced Europe could sustain another 500,000 deaths by next March. In Scotland, there has so far been no announcement. A further extension of the vaccine passport scheme is being mooted to embrace a wider range of venues but this is proving highly contentious.

23rd November

Boris at his most vacuous and buffoonish yesterday in a presentation to northern industrialists; losing command of his script and then veering off into a rambling disquisition on 'Peppa Pig'! He appears to be losing the plot. In addition, he has in the last fortnight successfully alienated not only his crony backbenchers in the South of England by raising the spectre of their having to relinquish their lucrative consultancies, but also the recently elected Tories in the North of England by cancelling much of the proposed rail extensions that were supposed to underpin the 'Northern Powerhouse'. Meanwhile, his so-called 'oven ready' plans for social care are giving the lie to the Government's avowed aims for 'levelling up'.

26th November

In more senses than one the calm before the storm. We are scheduled for Storm Arwen to hit us this evening with 60–70 mile-an-hour winds and possibly snow. Meanwhile, a new variant of the pandemic – B.1.1.129 named Omicron – has emerged from Southern Africa. It appears to have a higher infectivity rate than the Delta variant and more mutations, thus potentially able to outwit our existing vaccines. If it takes off in the UK this could certainly be a game changer and precipitate a new escalation in deaths and the reintroduction of stringent controls on our everyday lives. Significantly, the FTSE 100 dropped by 3.6%, the biggest fall in 18 months.

This week my mobility and balance has been markedly worse, and it is difficult not to despair of my condition. However, I have each day to remember that I need to enjoy and value the movement and functions that I do still have as they may not be there in a year's time. At least, sitting down, I can socialise quite normally and this week I much enjoyed our book group, and I am looking forward to having our cul-de-sac neighbours over for dinner tonight. I do still dearly miss not having a cat, but most of all I miss my wee Bella!

28th November

As I anticipated, the Omicron virus has now arrived in Britain and there is a distinct whiff of panic in Westminster with test and isolation controls and certain travel bans being reintroduced in England. Yet the Government is still maintaining a populist mantra of 'saving Christmas'. Nicola is keeping her options open but has heavily hinted that fresh controls may be required in addition to the masking and distancing regulations that are already in place.

The SNP ploughs blithely on with a finance minister who clearly lives in another world. Kate Forbes denies that Scotland has a deficit that would weigh down any form of independence. She constantly refers to any deficit as 'notional'. In fact, Scotland's deficit is estimated to be £36 billion for 2020–21; equivalent to 22.4% of GDP as compared with the UK at 14.2%.

We survived the storm without any damage. It is a miracle that the pyracantha has survived with its wonderful display of red berries on the front of the house. This morning sees the first snow of the winter – very scenic but likely to be treacherous once the ground refreezes. Hopefully this cold spell may attract some newcomers to the bird feeders. Tomorrow, Ella is due her appendix operation. I just hope all goes well and that the anomaly seen on a previous scan proves to be benign.

29th November

Predictably, there has been an outbreak of Omicron in the west of Scotland. It augurs badly for the Christmas festivities! At last, Keir Starmer appears to be getting a grip, and appointing some muscle to his shadow cabinet; in particular, Yvette Cooper as Shadow Home Secretary and David Lammy as Shadow Foreign Secretary. The Labour Party has been gifted so many open goals in the past two years and failed to capitalise on them. It desperately needs to formulate some constructive and properly costed policies if it ever going to appear a credible 'government in waiting'.

A new one for the lexicon – 'operationalise'– the latest government speak for 'implement', coined by a health spokesman in a tortured attempt to convey Government plans to expand the provision of booster vaccinations to all adults in England in response to the new variant. Just as a year ago, there is a worrying disconnect between the chummy festive optimism of Boris Johnson and the depressing reality of rising pandemic-related hospital admissions along with over 1,000 deaths a week and an escalating backlog in elective surgery. It remains to be seen how long another lockdown can be avoided.

6th December

The new variant is rapidly spreading in the UK and already new restrictions on travel are being imposed. Across Europe there is growing civil unrest against vaccination procedures and/ or fresh lockdowns with violent demonstrations in Austria and the Netherlands. As in the 19th century, the prospect of compulsory vaccination is highlighting the competing agendas of public health and civil liberties and the whole debate around the pandemic is being 'weaponised'.

Another storm (Barra) is due to hit us tomorrow adding yet another layer of impediment to our lives.

A better Parkinson's day yesterday. I managed to refill the feeders; a small task but important for my self-confidence. So far, no interesting visitors except a flock of long-tailed tits.

9th December

There is rising outrage at the evasive and duplicitous behaviour of the Prime Minister over the breaches of Covid restrictions last Christmas in the Cabinet Office. This, at a time when the Government is now imposing a new round of controls designed to contain the spread of the Omicron variant; a variant that appears to double the spread of infection every two to three days and threatens to become exponential. Coupled with the growing evidence of the inept and casual handling of the Afghanistan retreat by the Foreign Office, this Government appears to be steadily losing the support of even its own backbenchers.

11th December

Depressing news on the pandemic. The Omicron variant is now creating a further wave of infection and promising to create an unprecedented number of cases, predicted by the experts to be as many as one or two hundred thousand extra cases a day by the end of the month. Nicola has alerted us to the real possibility of a 'tsunami of infection' hitting the Scottish population in the coming weeks. Even if the existing vaccines prove able to reduce the severity of symptoms the sheer number of new cases will mean that the small proportion of cases requiring hospitalisation will still be large enough to overwhelm the NHS. In response, the Scottish Government have advised against any Christmas parties and other social gatherings for a second year, tightened up masking and testing requirements, and renewed its advice for people to work from home if possible. As yet another period of lockdown has not been imposed in an effort to minimise the damage to the economy and the mental health of the population, but all may change if Omicron realises our worst predictions. Meanwhile, the UK death rate from the pandemic continues to rise by around 1,000 per week and is now approaching 150,000!

14th December

A trip to Vane Farm yesterday to do some birdwatching. It was very cold but bracing. The scooter operated well but in one or two places the camber is dodgy. Unfortunately, the light was bad and it was difficult to identify the birds. Nothing special, just the usual suspects, predominantly widgeon and teal, with a good view of whooper swans and a hunting kestrel. As always, my tremor and bladder were a pain. I need to seriously rethink my clothing before I revisit the reserve and find a more efficient compromise between warmth and the need to access my privates!

15th December

We are now in a completely new ballgame with the pandemic. Cases of the Omicron variant are now rising exponentially and predicted to run into the millions in the immediate future. Medical experts view the situation as the worst scenario since the start of the pandemic. There is ever-increasing evidence that the NHS and Care sector are struggling to cope. The transmissibility of Omicron, with an R factor estimated as between 3 and 5, appears to far exceed that of the Delta variant, and its prevalence to be doubling every 1–2 days. Despite the best efforts of the swivel-eyed Tory libertarian backbenchers, the Government has been forced to legislate for a new round of controls and the First Minister has encouraged us to minimise all socialising over the Festive Season. My guess is that another lockdown is inevitable regardless of the collateral damage to the economy and the mental health of the population.

Thanks to Mo's efforts the Christmas tree looks great, but the house feels a little soul-less without my wee Bella!

18th December

This week has witnessed a massive by-election defeat for the Tories in North Shropshire and a growing discontent with Johnson's premiership in Westminster. His perpetual disregard of pandemic rules, defence of sleaze in Tory ranks, disrespect of industrial leaders, and vacuous responses to the legitimate concerns of the electorate, not to mention his unerring ability to bluster and lie, are happily being called to account.

As expected, the number of new Omicron cases continues to rise exponentially. At the same time, the resources of the health and care sectors are increasingly undermined by the number of staff forced to quarantine. The possibility of another lockdown, or in the current parlance, 'circuit break', is gaining increased support from medical experts and one wonders just what freedom of movement and socializing will still operate come Christmas Day!

Another neologism for the record: 'Quaranteenies', for the cohorts of teenagers who have had to endure the pandemic.

A sad remembrance day for mum who died in 1990 and for our little cat Zapher; such a character and so loved by all who met him. It is a low point of the year and one that I have always associated with grief over the death of family or pets or over the breakup of relationships. It is a struggle to remain positive.

Boxing Day

Everything feels very flat. The weather is dull and miserable and the rapid spread of Omicron has unravelled many of our plans for meeting up with friends. In effect, it is a modest lockdown but for now voluntarily imposed. Where we will be by the New Year heaven knows. I suppose the clearest indicator that all is again going belly-up will be an early recall of Parliament. On the Holyrood front the most notable development was the continued 'fiscal illiteracy' of Kate Forbes, the Scottish Cabinet Minister for Finance. She argued that the absence of the ability to use quantitative easing after independence to cope with any financial crisis was of little importance. Meanwhile, the incompetence of the SNP Government in furthering a green policy is increasingly evident. The SNP promised 130,000 new jobs in the renewable industries by 2020. In reality, only 20, 000 new jobs have been delivered, and the bulk of the manufacturing associated with the construction of offshore wind farms has been sourced abroad.

The usual cursory (20 minutes) appointment with my consultant. To minimise the hassle of a wholly inappropriate 9am appointment, I elected for a telephone session. As always there were no new medications in Dr D's armoury that he could recommend. However, he has suggested that I increase my dosage of Co-Careldopa in the hope of reducing my tremor.

29th December

The number of new Coronavirus cases per day is now exceeding 200,000 and rising. Hospital, care home, and transport sectors are struggling with an acute shortage of staff, either because they have become infected or because they have been forced to isolate as contacts. In anticipation that the situation will deteriorate, the NHS in England is establishing temporary Nightingale field stations (so-called 'surge hubs') in hospital grounds to house recovering patients so as to reduce the strain on hospital beds. The situation is further complicated by an acute shortage of lateral flow testing kits and delays in obtaining the results of PCR (polymerase chain reaction) tests. Yet, still the Government is refusing to impose more stringent controls until after the New Year in England in contrast to the more dirigiste stance of the devolved administrations. Intuitively, one feels that the future of Boris and his cronies will hinge on the course of the pandemic over the next ten days.

I have embarked on two new 'projects' to motivate me and give me some structure in 2022. First, I intend to improve my birdwatching and listening skills, and secondly, I intend to broaden the base of my academic expertise by reading all my back copies of the *Journal of the History of Sexuality*, of which I have a complete run.

A buzzard circling the conservatory today was a rare treat!

PART III

Living with the Virus 2022

5th January

A muted Hogmanay due to the pandemic with just a toast to the neighbours from our doorstep. For the first time we are beginning to hear of friends and relatives who have tested positive. Certainly, the festive season's plans of many have unravelled due to the infection. The number of new cases in the UK continues to rise, and with the return of students to schools and universities a further escalation in the prevalence of Omicron is anticipated. In England, Boris is continuing to hold back on additional restrictions despite many NHS trusts declaring that even non-Covid emergencies are being marginalised and patients encouraged to make their own way to A&E departments. The Government is trying to alleviate the serious loss of staff in the health, utility, and transport sectors by reducing the need in some circumstances for PCR tests and the length of self-isolation required of those testing positive, but this could mean infected people re-entering the labour force prematurely and merely spreading the variant still further.

Yesterday, we tried to take advantage of the sunny weather to get some fresh air for the sake of our mental health. Unfortunately, everyone else had the same idea and the car parks at Gullane Bents and Yellowcraigs were hoaching. It was far too cold for the scooter but just refreshing to see the sea and the windsurfers.

7th January

The front page of the *Scotsman* well captures the muddled priorities of the policy community, with declarations of intent to reopen the cultural life of the nation juxtaposed with the admission of the Scottish Health Secretary that the NHS is facing its biggest challenge in 73 years. It is estimated that one in twenty people in Scotland had Covid in the Christmas week and its prevalence continues to trend upwards. Notwithstanding Boris's boosterish assurances that we can ride out the current wave of infection, an increasing number of NHS trusts are declaring 'critical incidents' with the conjuncture of increased demand on emergency services and staff absences creating a perfect storm. All the while the vast backlog of elective surgery, not to mention routine primary care, is growing, and we have yet to confront the medical repercussions of long Covid that are only now becoming fully apparent.

15th January

An eventful week. Boris's position as PM seems increasingly precarious as evidence mounts of the disregard of Downing Street for pandemic restrictions during last year's lockdowns. Meanwhile, Prince Andrew has been shorn of his royal duties and honorary military posts and faces civil action for his alleged involvement in sexual abuse. All this is distracting from two areas of existential threat to our health and security: the likely invasion of Ukraine by Russia and the recurrence of pandemic outbreaks in China. My intuition is that a further, more virulent variant is lurking somewhere in the Far East. There has been a further loosening in travel and hospitality restrictions and in testing and self-isolating procedures despite daily recorded deaths from Covid in the UK regularly exceeding 350, and many millions estimated to be currently infected. It looks to me that the Cabinet has tacitly shifted back to the initial strategy of relying on 'herd immunity' to contain the pandemic, knowing that the elderly and vulnerable now have added protection from the booster vaccination. But it is a huge gamble that Boris and the

Tories are taking and if the current wave of infection fails to subside, they face being crucified in the coming local elections.

20th January

The policy community continues to exist on another planet from those at the front line of health and care provision. [Interestingly, the Care agencies also characterise the Government as inhabiting a 'parallel Universe'] Much of the test and isolation requirements are due to be relaxed or rescinded next week along with the mandatory wearing of masks. Official encouragement to work at home if possible is also being withdrawn. The official mantra is now that we must 'all get used to living with the virus', but it would be more accurate to say that 'we must also get used to dying from it'. Boris and Nicola both claim that we have ridden this third wave of infection and that it is projected to steadily diminish. This all assumes that another more virulent variant is not going to emerge: a brave assumption! Indeed, the World Health Organisation remains adamant that we are far from defeating the pandemic.

At Westminster, Boris continues to face calls for his resignation. David Davis, an erstwhile supporter of Boris, even resurrected Cromwell's injunction to the Long Parliament in 1653 and commanded Boris in the Commons: 'In the name of God go!' A new addition to our Covid lexicon: 'Red Meat'- meaning the sudden display of projected legislation by the Tory leadership, thrown out to placate the backbenchers and distract from the loss of public trust in the Government.

My Parkinson's has deteriorated again over the last month. My balance is worse, as is my tremor and agitation. I can no longer stay safe without a cane and the time has come when we need to investigate acquiring an indoor wheelchair. I am feeling distinctly off-colour at the moment, but my lateral flow test is negative.

30th. January

Two storms, (Malik and Corrie) have hit Scotland this weekend causing widespread damage and destruction. So far it appears that the house and garden are intact – even the pyracantha! Fortunately, Paul and I were able to visit Vane Farm on Friday before the weather fully closed in. However, with the wind chill, the temperature was positively Baltic. As on our previous visit, the light was poor, but we had a brilliant sighting of whooper swans along with the usual suspects – teal, widgeon, golden eye, tufted duck, mallard, and a welcome group of curlew. The scooter worked well and by taking a different route to the third hide we were able to avoid the dodgy camber on the path down to the first hide.

The week's politics have been surreal. Faced with the real prospect of war in Ukraine and social unrest at home due to a dramatic increase in the cost of living (especially a crippling rise in fuel costs), the Government has been totally distracted by the ongoing furore over the breaching of Covid regulations by Downing Street during the lockdown over the 2020 festive season (so-called 'Partygate'). Boris's tenure as PM hangs in the balance.

Today, in accordance with my consultant's advice, I have increased my Co-careldopa medication to see if it can reduce my tremor. I suspect, to begin with, it will make me feel light-headed, but it is worth a try. With the relaxation of pandemic restrictions NHS Scotland has offered me a yellow lanyard or badge to alert others that I still need people to distance themselves given that I am categorised as especially vulnerable. I doubt that I will take up the offer. My intuition is that before long another variant will emerge, and the restrictions will be re-imposed.

7th February

Not a good start to the week. Feeling faint and having to lie down. I suspect it is due to low blood pressure related to mixing Co-careldopa with my breakfast. I need to start taking my tablets on an empty stomach. I suspect there may also be some inner ear issues as I have not had them treated for several years due to the pandemic. I have been spending more time on listening to bird song CDs and watching winter watch on TV. I find this calming and it resets my recognition skills for the new year. At the moment the weather is either too cold or too windy to venture out on my scooter, but I must get out of the house more, even if it is just to walk around the garden.

We had a really enjoyable Zoom with Canada yesterday. Clearly, they are struggling with the pandemic again. There is disturbing news from Ottawa where truck drivers have effectively shut down the city centre in protest at Covid restrictions. The situation is so bad that a state of emergency has been called. Worryingly, there are strong echoes of the attack on the US Capitol with civil unrest being fuelled by professional agitators with rabid right-wing agendas.

At home, Boris is still clinging on for all he is worth despite the resignation of virtually all his Downing Street team. Meanwhile, our First Minister seems to be adopting an increasingly fractious style at Holyrood. Her latest proposals with respect to school pandemic arrangements are worthy of the Mad Hatter's Tea Party. At the very moment that the Scottish executive is imposing the legal requirement for all premises to have an integrated alarm system she is recommending that all schools should shave the base off their doors so as ensure ventilation, contrary to the most basic fire regulations!

14th February

War in Ukraine is threatened, and many observers anticipate an imminent Russian invasion. The situation is being described as the most serious threat since the Cuban missile crisis. Should Putin move his troops into Ukraine, the US and NATO threaten to impose a range of crippling trade and financial sanctions on Russia. Peculiarly, my main concern has not been the prospect of war but the fact that Boris and his self-serving cronies will use it to distract the British public from their egregious behaviour during lockdown. It is a measure of how this Government has distorted our priorities.

A major divergence between the Covid policies in England and Scotland is emerging. In England, it is proposed that all mandatory restrictions relating to distancing, masking, testing, and isolating should be removed at the end of February. Much to the disquiet of many medical experts and NHS managers, and contrary to the advice of the WHO, people who test positive will no longer be legally required to isolate south of the Border. In effect, the Government is advocating that we must get used to 'living with the Covid virus' for the foreseeable future even if a more laissez faire policy leads to a further escalation in the level of infections. However, Scotland is maintaining its policy of 'test and isolate'. It is all becoming very messy and much to do with political manoeuvring on Boris's part. Certainly, there has been no effort to disclose the 'science' behind this latest change of policy.

My increased dosage of Careldopa has left me feeling very light-headed and faint. The symptoms appear to be worse if I take the tablets on an empty stomach. Otherwise, my disturbed sleep pattern continues as before. Watching Carole King last night brought back so many memories and regrets of opportunities squandered 40 years ago: demons that will haunt me all my life.

But as they say, 'That way madness lies', and I must live in the present!

The weather is about to present us with yet another challenge, with storms Dudley and Eunice due to hit us later in the week with winds up to 70mph.

Ps I spotted a lovely pair of long-tailed tits on the replenished feeders today.

PPs I later came across a sentence in a book I was reading for our Book Group that really moved me and shone a more positive light on my regrets: 'It is only our heartaches that finally refutes all that is ephemeral in love.'

17th February

It appears that we have survived storm Dudley intact and there are indications that Eunice will centre more in England. I had another Zoom last night with my former Parentline colleagues. The profile of callers to the help line has shifted with an increasing focus on monetary issues. The impact on poorer families of the rise in the cost of living is fast becoming a major concern. The consumer price index inflation reached 5.3% in January, the highest level since 1992, and is predicted to rise to well over 7% by March. Fuel costs have risen exponentially, and the level of fuel poverty is unprecedented. It appears that the Bank of England will have to raise bank rate in order to try and curb inflation. However, this in turn will have a serious impact on all those who acquired loans and mortgages in recent years at favourable interest rates, as well as inflating the interest accruing on the national debt incurred during the pandemic. Yet another perfect storm!

20ᵗʰ February

Boris has warned that we are on the brink of the biggest war in Europe since the Second World War. I just wish I could repress my cynicism that he is deliberately playing to a Churchillian narrative as a means of distracting us from the consequences of 'Partygate'.

Storm Eunice passed through with little damage here but, in Suffolk, my brother has clearly been severely impacted with extensive damage to his gates and fencing. With another storm (Franklin) scheduled for tomorrow, there is every likelihood of more flooding and destruction down South. So far, the threat of snowfall in Scotland has not been realised in the Dalkeith area but other parts of Scotland have experienced blizzards and power outages.

22ⁿᵈ February

Putin has today effectively invaded Ukraine by recognising the rebel-held regions in Eastern Ukraine as independent sovereign republics and moving Russian troops into the area. The USA and EU are responding with heavy financial and economic sanctions. The situation is fraught and all hangs on whether Putin authorises further military advances.

Perhaps it is an omen that today is the last palindrome date for many years - 22/02/2022!

Today, the First Minister has announced that she anticipates all legal Covid restrictions will be removed by the third week of March, with some requirements, such as the use of vaccine passports at hospitality and other venues, becoming voluntary as of next week. However, Nicola is determined to retain test and isolate procedures with free lateral flow kits for the foreseeable future, irrespective of Boris's initiatives; the funding for which has become yet another point of friction with the Treasury. With waiting times at A&E at their worst since last January, one cannot but feel that this is 'all going to end in tears'.

24th February

Today, Europe is again at war! Putin has authorised the full-scale invasion of Ukraine. Fighting has already begun, and the military offensive is backed by cyber-attacks. This threatens to be a watershed moment in the geopolitical history of the continent. All the usual collateral effects on money markets are evident with the FTSE currently down by almost 3%. In addition, the price of oil is escalating with the prospect of acute supply constraints given that Russia is the second largest exporter of oil.

28th February

The news from Ukraine is bleak and utterly depressing with scenes all too reminiscent of the Second World War in Europe. Quite apart from the heart-breaking impact on the lives of the Ukrainians, the economic fall-out from sanctions is likely to affect all of us as consumers. It will be interesting to see how far the map of Europe will have altered in six months' time.

29th February

Putin has put his nuclear forces on alert and the EU has authorised and funded the provision of armaments to Ukraine. The situation remains critical. Ukrainian fighters have so far put up a stiff resistance, but Putin may well launch another more vicious offensive. At home, Priti Patel continues to display a callous disregard for the plight of migrants, insisting on maintaining restrictive and protracted visa controls on Ukrainian refugees (already numbering half a million), unlike the open-door response of many European countries. Not only has this Government no ethics, it has no soul! Meanwhile, the value of the Russian rouble has plunged by 30% and the Russian banking system is virtually paralysed. We would be naïf to assume that we will be immune from the economic repercussions of our sanctions, but sometimes repelling evil and injustice comes at a cost. Sadly, our Foreign Secretary is out of her depth and a complete lightweight.

3rd March

The situation in Ukraine is unbearably sad and has eclipsed all the other issues including 'Partygate', the pandemic, and the rising cost of living. The Russian invasion has been protracted due in no small part to the heroic resistance from the Ukrainian forces and civilians. Sadly, this slow progress of the invasion may incur greater destruction and casualties than if the take-over had been swift and decisive. Already, many thousands of Ukrainians have been killed and to date around one million have fled to other neighbouring countries. It seems likely that war crimes have been committed with Russian troops targeting civilians and using cluster bombs and thermobaric weapons. A massive convoy of armour is slowly approaching Kyiv. At the moment it appears to be suffering logistical problems, but it is undoubtedly about to lay siege to the city.

Meanwhile, although the US and EU are supplying arms to the Ukrainian defence forces, they are not prepared to try and introduce a no-fly zone for fear of precipitating a Third World War. Many military experts feel that Putin has miscalculated and that in the medium to long term he will be displaced. However, in the short term the outcome of this deadly episode will remain primarily in his murderous hands.

5th March

The war in Ukraine has now become an existential threat to the whole continent with the Russian army firing on the biggest nuclear plant in Europe. Fortunately, the building encasing the rods was not hit but the situation remains hazardous, especially if the invasion cuts off the means of cooling the rods as happened in Chernobyl. Meanwhile, the Russian army is systematically reducing the towns and cities of Ukraine to rubble and creating an exodus of biblical proportions. Some military experts are predicting that, if the war becomes protracted and Putin adopts 'siege' tactics, he might even resort to using chemical and/or biological weapons, as in Syria. The whole episode is further deepening our mood, already at a low ebb with Brexit, the pandemic, and the imminent threat of IndyRef2.

8th March

The news from Ukraine is heart-breaking. After thirteen days of conflict Ukraine is fast becoming a humanitarian disaster area. Thousands of innocent civilians are besieged in towns and cities without food, water, and medical supplies, in subfreezing temperatures, while subject to a constant barrage of shelling. The Red Cross has described the living conditions of the population as 'apocalyptic'. Many civilians have been killed or injured in the fighting or have died through hypothermia or dehydration. To add to their misery every attempt to create 'humanitarian corridors' to allow the population to safely relocate has proved abortive.

Meanwhile, Priti Patel has once again proved herself to be unfit for office, blithely announcing a more liberal immigration procedure for Ukrainian refugees while still requiring them to obtain a barometric test and a visa in Paris or Brussels before entry from Calais! To date less than 800 applications for entry into the UK have been processed at a time when countries such as Poland, Czechoslovakia, and Germany have already welcomed tens of thousands of refugees (in Poland's case well over a million) fleeing across the borders of Ukraine. The tabloids aptly dismissed the Home Office's dismal performance as 'Priti Pathetic'.

There is continuing concern over the interference of the invading forces with the operation of the nuclear plants and, ominously, the prospect of a Third World War has become part of the narrative. Certainly, the sanctions currently being imposed will have global implications for fuel and food supplies, and the resulting rise in prices and the cost of living will almost certainly lead to increased levels of poverty and deprivation across the world.

Amidst the international crisis there remains the ever-present threat of the pandemic. Covid-19 legal restrictions are being eased in Scotland. Businesses and event organisers are no longer legally required to ask for proof of vaccination. People will no longer legally have to wear face coverings in public and hospitality venues will no longer have to collect customer details for contact tracing. However, everyone is encouraged to continue to take basic precautions and to do a lateral flow test at least twice a week or before meeting someone from a 'high risk' group. Should the test prove positive, contrary to new procedures south of the Border, the Scottish guidelines stress that you should still go for a PCR test. Curiously though, there is no mention of a need to isolate. The most interesting departure is a review of the 'Highest Risk List'. Given the success of the vaccination programme and the introduction of new treatments for those contracting the Coronavirus, the previous 'shielded' list is likely to be drastically reduced. Whether my 'shielded' days are over remains to be seen.

Yesterday, a delightful and moving few minutes overlooking the sea at Longniddry Bents listening to a choir singing for the people of Ukraine. We will need many more such healing moments in the coming days.

13th March

News from Ukraine and from Covid-19 is bleak. Russian troops are laying siege to a whole range of towns and cities and closing in on Kyiv.

Meanwhile, some virologists have detected a new Deltacron Corona variant circulating in France, the US, the Netherlands and Denmark that is beginning to ring alarm bells. This is especially so as, according to the UK Health Security Agency, the number of elderly people contracting Covid and requiring hospital treatment is on the increase. In Scotland the level of Covid infections was at its highest last week since the pandemic began; some 300,000 or one in sixteen people.

16th March

The narrative around Ukraine is increasingly seen as akin to Germany's invasion of Poland in 1939 or the Spanish Civil War, with the real prospect of a continental and thereby a World War. China is aligning itself, albeit cautiously, with Putin, and some international observers are predicting that it may take the opportunity, with the distraction of Ukraine, to invade Taiwan. Meanwhile, there is a continuing concern over the safety of the nuclear plants in Ukraine.

The war in Ukraine and the severe sanctions imposed by the Western allies are having a drastic effect on world commodity and fuel prices. Inflation in the UK is nearing 9% while average wage increases are estimated to have risen by only 3.7%, fuelling low-income deprivation and the prospect of industrial unrest. And, with all this taking centre stage, there is the danger that we will lose traction on the pandemic.

19th March

Significantly, Sturgeon has retained for another month the legal requirements for masking in Scotland in view of the rising incidence of BA.2 in Scotland.

Yesterday, I enjoyed another visit to Vane Farm with PS. We missed our bacon butties as the café was closed but saw a fair range of birds including greylag and pink-footed geese, widgeon, teal, gadwall, golden eye, tufted duck, pochard, and a splendid sight of lapwings.

21st March

It is now two years since I first kept this diary. In many ways life has barely changed since the first lockdown. The pandemic, now with a new, highly contagious variant- Omicron BA.2- is still a dominant feature in our lives. Although many of the previous restrictions are now being relaxed, today's *Scotsman* reports that the number of Covid patients in Scottish hospitals is at an all-time high and several Health Trusts are again fearful of being overwhelmed. Meanwhile, the campaign to oust Johnson for his egregious behaviour has been overshadowed by events in Ukraine where Putin's siege warfare is threatening to escalate, with the use of chemical and possibly nuclear weapons triggering a potentially apocalyptic war with NATO. Already it is calculated that 10 million people have been displaced with harrowing scenes reminiscent of the Second World War.

We spent last weekend at Crieff Hydro. As usual, everyone was hugely supportive. The weather for once was fine and the views en route truly outstanding. Gayle and the twins were with us and watching them in the evenings with the magician and dancing to the ceilidh band was delightful.

Thanks to Mo we have made some real progress with our plans for my 80th and dates have now been fixed for a family do and a larger event at Howies for my wider group of friends later in the summer. But before then Mo has to contend with her dental surgery and I have to keep upright and out of hospital! Weather permitting, I am hoping to spend a good deal of time in the garden. With Hilary's help I want to revive the wee pond and put some fish in it. Martin is also going to modify some of the paving so that I can access the garden with my scooter.

24th March

Yesterday we spent an idyllic afternoon at Gosford Estate soaking up some much-needed sun. It was unseasonably warm with no wind and very peaceful except for the occasional honks of the greylag geese and other birdsong including nuthatch, woodpecker, and chiff chaff.

The Chancellor's Spring Statement did very little to address the rising cost of living crisis. The Office for Budget Responsibility has calculated that this year will see the biggest drop in family disposable incomes since the 1950s. Inflation is widely anticipated to rise to 9% and the level of taxation is at an historic high. Predicted annual growth of GDP has been revised down from 6% to a mere 3.8%. The overall effect of Rishi Sunak's mini budget is regressive, with no mention of a windfall tax on the profits of oil and gas companies who are making excessive profits out of the fuel price hikes. 'Levelling Up' remains a chimera!

Today marks a month since Ukraine was invaded. There are indications that in some areas Russian troops are being forced to retreat but this may merely encourage Putin to deploy chemical or even nuclear weapons.

27th March

It is estimated that one in eleven people in Scotland now have the Omicron virus (predominantly the BA.2 sub-variant) and according to the latest official modelling, the number infected every day could reach 60,000 by mid-April. While this may not feed through to any dramatic increase in the need for intensive care, it will impact on hospital beds and frustrate any significant improvement in reducing the backlog in elective surgery. In addition, the increase in hospital admissions and Covid-related staff shortages are creating ever-growing delays in A&E departments, often leading to avoidable deaths.

Worrying signs that Biden is straying dangerously from his script. Twice this week he has made comments which Putin could easily exploit, and which misrepresented the policy of the western allies. On the issue of the use of chemical weapons in Ukraine, he threatened to retaliate 'in kind'. He also remarked that Putin was 'a butcher': adding, 'For God's sake this man cannot remain in power', thus suggesting that the US is seeking 'regime change' in Russia. The White House subsequently sought to add a gloss to these statements but Biden has a reputation for making gaffs and this may all cost him dearly in the mid-term elections.

At home, the Chancellor's Spring Statement has attracted widespread criticism for failing to address properly the cost-of-living crisis. The optics suggested that he was more concerned with enhancing his image as a potential leader, than engaging with the prospect of a dramatic increase in social deprivation in the coming months. The Resolution Foundation, an independent think-tank, estimates that some 1.3 million people in the United Kingdom will be driven into poverty over the coming months.

The weather has been beautiful this week and it has been a joy to bask in the sun in the garden. Mo is due to go to Cellardyke next weekend and this will be a good test of my coping on my own.

31st March

The weather is fickle. After a week of unseasonably warm days, we now have 'thunder snow' and sub-zero winds from the north. Certainly, it is too cold for using the scooter but hopefully on Sunday Hilary and Martin will be able to take me down the east coast for some casual birdwatching from the car. A poor dental day with gingivitis and a cracked tooth being diagnosed, at a predicted treatment cost of £300.

The situation in Ukraine is complex. Putin seems to have at last accepted that his anticipation of a speedy invasion was misplaced and he is now intending to focus his troops in Eastern Ukraine. There is some evidence that the Russian troops are demoralised and even abandoning their weaponry in some areas. However, in other places the systematic destruction of the country's infrastructure continues along with the indiscriminate targeting of civilian communities. It is hoped that, at last, the estimated 140,000 people still surviving in dire conditions in Mariupol may be rescued today by a convoy of Red Cross evacuation buses during a temporary truce. The city has become a 'humanitarian catastrophe' and, like Grozny and Odessa, has become defined by its total devastation. For the moment, the attack on Kyiv appears to have temporarily stalled but military observers warn that once the invasion force has regrouped and re-equipped, the real battle for the capital may begin.

2nd April

A day of bleak news. The planned evacuation of Mariupol was again aborted as sufficient guarantees of safe passage could not be obtained from the Russians. So, yet one more day for the Ukrainian inhabitants trapped for over a month without food, water, heating, and medical supplies, with bodies lying in the streets.

At home, the level of Covid infections continues at an historic high with one in thirteen people in the UK population – some 5 million – thought to have succumbed to the second wave (BA.2) of the Omicron virus. The number of hospitalisations and deaths has also risen. Perversely, the Government is intent on dismantling the 'test and trace' system and free lateral flow tests are being phased out contrary to the advice of some leading epidemiologists. There appears to have been a shift in the narrative surrounding the pandemic towards an acceptance that we just have to learn to live with it while protecting the vulnerable. However, such a view fails to take account of the scale of absenteeism in the NHS and care sector that such a level of infection will create.

Mo has gone away for a short break to Fife and I am acutely aware of how much I now depend on her. Even the smallest tasks are taking an age given my lack of balance and scrambled footwork.

4th April

Yesterday, Hilary and Martin took me out to East Lothian for a picnic and some birdwatching. Unfortunately, the tide was out and, apart from a goldeneye at Musselburgh and an eider at Longniddry Bents, there was little to see. However, it was clear that my best bet in the future is Musselburgh along the mouth of the Esk as long as the tides are right.

Appalling news today of war crimes in Ukraine carried out by Russian troops as they retreated East from Kyiv, including rape and the systematic shooting of civilians.

7th April

The situation in Ukraine remains dire. Although the Russian troops are withdrawing to the East in order to secure the region of the Donbas, they are leaving devastation in their wake. Their retreat is littered with civilian corpses and stories of the indiscriminate killing, rape and mutilation of Ukrainians. Mariupol has been described as a 'graveyard'. Many military experts predict that the main battle will be in the Donbas and that it will involve a level of engagement not seen since the Second World War. Meanwhile, the inability of the Home Office to create a fast entry process to the UK for Ukrainian refugees is a disgrace. As of today, only 15% of those applying for entry visas have been processed. There is also concerning evidence that in order to try and address mounting criticism, the Home Office has been de-prioritising Afghan cases.

A range of other contentious issues is questioning the Government's competence and integrity. Although the war in Ukraine may for the moment have diverted attention away from 'Partygate', it has not gone away. The news today that the Chancellor's wife has non-dom tax status, at a time when the public is facing a dramatic rise in the cost of living and increased national insurance contributions, merely adds to the prevailing impression of sleaze and hypocrisy in the ruling elite. Meanwhile, the Government has barely addressed the existential threat to low-income families of the rise in food and fuel prices.

I have been listening to a wonderful series of podcasts by Alistair Campbell and Rory Stewart: *The Rest is Politics.* Listening to Rory reflecting on current events really brings home the lack of intellectual rigour and moral compass in the current Government.

My walking indoors goes from bad to worse and my freezing and agitation get no better. I have therefore made a phone appointment with my GP to see if I can get some form of tranquillizer to take the edge off my stress. This would greatly improve my quality of life and enable me to venture out more. I also have my second booster next week. In addition, Martin has created a ramp down into the garden that will enable me to use the scooter around the garden when the weather improves and the grass firms up. I might even be able to do the watering from it!

8th April

Today we purchased an indoor wheelchair to facilitate my moving around the house. Sad that my mobility issues have come to this, but it is probably wise to be proactive.

13th April

I had my second booster jab two days ago with the Moderna vaccine. Yesterday I was feeling washed out with sore muscles and a slight temperature, and I had to retire to bed in the morning. However, I was better by the end of the day and slept well.

The Ukraine situation threatens to precipitate a major war. Putin is determined to regain the east of Ukraine at the very least and is prepared to devastate the area if necessary. Meanwhile, NATO has ramped up the supply of so-called 'defensive weapons' to the Ukrainians including anti-tank and anti-aircraft missiles. It seems only a matter of time before direct confrontation is triggered. In the light of the stories told by those fleeing from Mariupo, where it is estimated that more than 20,000 people have been killed, including over 10,000 civilians, Biden has begun to accuse Putin of ethnic cleansing.

Here at home, 'Partygate' has returned with a vengeance. Both the Prime Minister and Chancellor have been fined for contravening the lockdown rules along with many others in the Downing Street bubble. But it appears that neither Johnson nor Sunak is prepared to resign, their supporters arguing that it would be inappropriate to initiate a new leadership contest or ministerial reshuffle when the Ukraine and the cost-of- living crisis deserve their undivided attention. Political commentators reckon that they will survive in the short term but, in the medium term, a lot will hinge on the outcome of the forthcoming local elections.

Meanwhile, it is difficult to believe that the UK is one of the wealthiest societies in the world. The incidence of poverty is rising exponentially with the dramatic rise in food and fuel prices, and any increase in family incomes being more than offset by rising inflation, which pre-pandemic was a mere 0.7% and is now projected to be near 9%. Travel is also becoming a nightmare with huge delays at the airports due to shortage of border control staff. In addition, it is utter mayhem at Dover due to the withdrawal of P&O ferries for safety checks, occasioned by the egregious sacking of all the existing crews in order to employ cheaper labour.

14th April

Yet another 'Mad Hatter's Tea Party' courtesy of Priti Patel. She is now proposing to fly to Rwanda all migrants illegally crossing the channel, to be processed in Rwanda with a view to their settling in Africa!! Oblivious to the irony, she has christened this monstrous enterprise a 'Migration and Economic Development Partnership'. The lack of empathy revealed in this scheme is breath-taking, as is its total disregard for human rights. I hope it buries her political career. The 'optics' surrounding the Government's current behaviour are toxic. Only the fortuitous opportunity for Boris to play the statesman occasioned by the Ukrainian war has enabled him to survive in post.

17th April

Another highly enjoyable afternoon in the peaceful surroundings of Gosford Park. Given that it is the Easter weekend, it was remarkably quiet. Still no sign of all the herons, but lovely to see the little grebe.

Predictably, Priti Patel's Rwandan 'folly' has caused a furore. Significantly, she has been forced to issue a Ministerial Directive, a seldom-used device, so as to overrule any objections from her civil servants. I suspect this will become a major issue of contention in the Commons when it reconvenes next week. The scheme has already been condemned by the UNHCR and the Archbishop of Canterbury.

In Ukraine, in response to the sinking of the Russians' Black Sea flagship, Kyiv has been heavily targeted by long-range missiles. Elsewhere, sadly it appears likely that Mariupol will soon be lost to the Russian invaders with a dire future in prospect for the thousands of Ukrainians who have not been able or willing to leave the city. The US and NATO are now furnishing Zelensky with a fresh supply of heavy weapons, but ominously Putin has warned that this may lead, in his words, to *'unpredictable consequences'*.

The drift of French politics also threatens the geopolitical stability of Western Europe should Marine le Pen become President after the second round of elections. Like Victor Orbán in Hungary she will bring to French politics the worst form of racist xenophobia and undermine the unity of the European Union and NATO in her obsession with national identity.

23rd April

An arduous week spending an hour each day scraping the driveway clean. Oddly enough, I am able to keep my balance for an hour even if I am stumbling indoors. I have started to practise on my new indoor wheelchair. It is more difficult than it looks to negotiate from one room to another without chipping the woodwork, but it is a sporty wee thing, and I am sure I will value it in the future. I also had my bloods checked as part of an annual review by the General Practice. Hopefully, nothing sinister will emerge.

'Partygate' continues its relentless course. The main development this week is that Johnson is to be investigated by an all-party committee to establish whether or not he has lied to the House. It appears that his tactic of delaying proceedings in the hope that the issue will go away has signally failed and, if anything, Tory backbench opinion is hardening against him. Certainly, he is mincemeat if the Tories suffer in the local elections.

The situation in the Ukraine remains dire with the Ukrainian army still holding out in Mariupol in the steel plant. A great deal will hinge on how quickly NATO can facilitate the supply of heavy armour and missiles to the Ukrainians without precipitating an apocalyptic response from Putin. Meanwhile, the UN Human Rights Monitoring Commission is uncovering a 'horror story of violations' and mass graves in territory recently abandoned by Russian troops. The war is also having an increasing impact on world markets and threatening to create food shortages and starvation in lesser-developed economies.

Happily, all those invited to my 80th birthday dinner party on 4th August at Howies, are able to come. I feel very privileged.

I received from Andy a digitised version of the ancestry work Dad did in his retirement. This will give me plenty of leads when I start my own research in the fall, when, if all goes well, I may have a little furry fellow to keep me company. Andy and Charlene have two adorable Bengal kittens (at I imagine a considerable price), and I do miss the calming presence of a 'cat on lap'.

Not a great deal of birdlife at the moment. A few of the usual suspects on the feeders plus a goldfinch and long-tailed tits on the wing and the distinctive piping of oyster catchers flying over. I also thought I heard the mewing of a buzzard circling somewhere overhead this afternoon.

28th April

A visit from an old St Catharine's College friend, today. He has lived a very full and fascinating, if somewhat tortured life. Despite a range of afflictions, including PTSD (from his time colluding with the ANC in Southern Africa and nurturing LGBT groups in Zimbabwe) and occasional bouts of ME, he still maintains a hectic schedule of travel and ministry. He brought back many memories of our survival in college in the freezing cold of the winter of 1961–2.

The narrative of Tory sleaze gains yet more momentum. A furious debate has surrounded the reported allegations of some Tory backbenchers that Angela Rayner deliberately performs a 'Sharon Stone' in the Chamber to distract Boris Johnson! A further furore surrounds the claim that a Tory MP was watching pornography in the Chamber. With the outcome of various 'Partygate' investigations still to come, Boris looks increasingly embattled, or will he do a 'Trump' and emerge undamaged in the local elections, the electorate having already accepted as normal the outrageous behaviour of the Prime Minister and his sleazy confidants.

The situation in Ukraine looks ominously as though it is drifting into total war with the ever-present threat of nuclear disaster. Liz Truss has now argued for NATO to facilitate the provision of fighter planes to the Ukrainians. Moreover, she has redefined the military objectives as removing the Russian troops from the whole of Ukraine including the territory occupied by Putin in 2014. In response, Putin has put Russia's nuclear deterrent forces on high alert!

30ᵗʰ April

'Porngate' has now been added to 'Partygate' and 'Pestminster' is another neologism in the tabloid press.

As of the end of May the Highest Risk List employed during the pandemic will close on the grounds that with the vaccines and new medications the most vulnerable are far less likely to be seriously ill with Covid. In a way it is a watershed moment as I will no longer be officially 'shielded' after over two years. At the same time, the test, trace, and isolate procedures are being wound down and the prescriptive aspects of the management of the pandemic are effectively abandoned. Interestingly, the pandemic has ceased to be a leading issue on the news and government spokesmen have begun to mention it in the past tense. Sadly, my balance and mobility have deteriorated so much that I doubt that all this will make a great deal of difference to my social life.

7ᵗʰ May

On Tuesday we celebrated our 25ᵗʰ wedding anniversary. Such fond memories of our stay at the Selkirk Arms and the ceremony in Gatehouse of Fleet. We arrived on the day after the New Labour landslide election victory in 1997. Little did we know that all the euphoria surrounding the result would eventually dissipate and let the Tories back in again. I firmly believed they were permanently injured as a political force.

Today we have the results of local elections in the UK. So far, as predicted, the Tory Party has suffered a considerable, but not cataclysmic, loss of seats. Labour has gained some notable seats in London but does not appear to have regained any traction in the Midlands and North of England. This has partly been seen as a hangover from the last general election and a persisting distrust of the Labour left, newly christened by Laura Kuenssberg as 'long Cobyn'. Meanwhile, the Liberal Democrats and Green Party have both made considerable gains. However, there are many seats still to be declared especially in Scotland and Northern Ireland where counting has only begun today. The Scottish result will have important implications for the SNP's campaign for Scottish independence while the prospect of a Sinn Fein majority promises to create a dramatic step-change in the political make-up of Northern Ireland.

Yesterday's economic predictions of the Bank of England are dire. It anticipates negative growth and possibly recession in 2023 accompanied by inflation at 10 percent. Bank rate was raised to 1% and further increases were expected.

13th May

I have now received a letter from the CMO confirming that my 'shielded' status is officially closed as of 31st May and that, as a fully vaccinated person, there is now 'no need to avoid contact'. It does however urge everyone to continue to wear a face covering in public places and on transport. It all sounds a bit inconsistent.

I am busy reading *The History Man* for our book group. A splendid read, laying bare the pretensions of late twentieth-century social scientists and the tortuous personal and professional interactions of university life. It contains some hilarious vignettes along with a vicious exposé of emotional and academic abuse.

17th May

Very warm weather today and it was a pleasure to soak up some sun in the garden. However, my balance and mobility are dire, and I even froze completely when faced with the modest slope into the garden created by Martin. The variation in my condition from day to day is a mystery and it is very disheartening. I might get the physiotherapist to observe me and see if she can improve my balance and motion. Certainly, her advice about my neck has made a real difference.

Everything feels a bit flat. The pandemic has not gone away but it has now become normalised and drifted from front-page news in favour of an outbreak of Monkey Pox in England. What perhaps deserves closer attention is the exponential spread of Omicron infections in North Korea, which, given its lack of vaccinations, is a prime breeding ground for a new variant!

Ukraine continues to occupy the media. In some areas the Russians have been driven back to their borders, but it appears as though it is going to be a long-drawn out struggle, most probably with an unsatisfactory compromise peace at the end. In the meantime, Sweden and Finland have elected to join NATO, which is the polar opposite of Putin's initial aims. In contrast, Johnson and Truss are further alienating the EU, and forfeiting what little trust international opinion still has in Britain, by threatening to overturn the Northern Ireland Protocol. Moreover, if they proceed in this regard, they will severely undermine their chances of securing a free trade agreement with the USA which views the Protocol as vital to the preservation of the Good Friday Peace Agreement. Needless to say, 'Partygate' still hovers in the background and continues to divert the Westminster bubble from the real issues of the day; in particular the impending 'apocalyptic' [the word used by the head of the Bank of England] rise in the cost of living with inflation at a forty-year high and heading for 'double-digits'.

20th May

It beggars belief!! While the Metropolitan Police have issued 126 fixed penalty notices for the breach of Covid restrictions in and around Downing Street in 2020, Boris Johnson has received only ONE. It defies logic that he attended a series of gatherings deemed to have breached the rules without himself being fined. However, Sue Gray's forthcoming report will hopefully prove far more damning. It will be a tragic irony if after all the egregious behaviour surrounding 'Partygate', Johnson survives in Office but the Durham Police fine Keir Starmer, and he has to step down from the Labour leadership.

25th May

Sue Gray's report has now been published. It is an excoriating account of the culture in Downing Street during the worst of the pandemic and the lack of leadership. Unfortunately, it does not precisely attribute blame to Boris and it looks as though he will survive, though his reputation will have been seriously scarred.

Meanwhile, the unrelenting rise in the cost of living is creating widespread poverty and unrest. The energy price-cap for October is projected to increase by 42% to £2,800, driving millions of people into 'fuel poverty'.

On Monday, PS and I had our monthly visit to Vane Farm. The light was excellent and we managed to see well over 20 species. The bonus was a close sighting of a reed bunting.

Today, Mo has had her major dental surgery lasting many hours. Unfortunately, due to the difficulty in finding a vein, sedation was not possible, so they have had to work with diazepam and local anaesthetic. Hilary has been a godsend, ferrying Mo to and from the surgery and helping me at home.

30th May

Mo is recovering well from her ordeal. Her face is still puffy and her lips badly blistered but so far the painkillers seem to have proved effective. Over the weekend we heard the wonderful news that Gayle had been awarded a Personal Chair in the History of Medicine. As my former doctoral student, post-doctoral research associate, faculty colleague, and co-author, but above all our dearest friend and 'surrogate daughter', her promotion means so much to us. We are so proud of her.

Predictably, the Sue Gray report on 'Partygate' let Boris off the hook. Effectively, the Metropolitan Police neutered the case against him and helped delay the proceedings long enough for any Tory backbench revolt to dissipate. It is also highly likely that pressure was put on Sue Gray to modify the final version of her report. The whole episode has severely compromised the public's faith in, and respect for, the British political system. Hopefully, the forthcoming by-elections will demonstrate the collateral damage inflicted on the Tory Party by Johnson's egregious behaviour.

A bad Parkinson's day yesterday with very little stability. I had to devolve the watering of the garden to Mo; one job I had hoped to continue. However, I need to reconcile myself to the fact that no two days are the same and go with the moment.

4th June

101 days since Putin invaded Ukraine. Sadly, it appears as though it is going to be a protracted war of attrition with little prospect in the near future of anyone suing for peace. The more the Russian troops advance, the heavier and more sophisticated the weapons

supplied by NATO to the Ukrainians. As a result, military experts are not anticipating any decisive outcome of hostilities. Indeed, it is difficult to conceive of any viable peace settlement. Meanwhile, the impact of the war on the production and distribution of grain, wheat, and fertilizer, and on world food prices, is threatening a global humanitarian disaster.

At home we are now in the third of four days celebration of the 70 years of Elizabeth's reign – her Platinum Jubilee. I personally have no interest in the proceedings and still less in the endless stream of sycophantic programmes aired on the BBC.

I am increasingly frustrated by my lack of mobility. There is less and less I can accomplish, and everything is so time-consuming. Yesterday, I calculated that it took me four solid hours to get myself up, showered and dressed, and breakfasted. However, on a more positive note, taking a diazepam clearly takes the edge of my agitation when I have commitments away from home. It worked a treat at the dentists and will clearly be a godsend in August when we go to Howies for my 80th and to Ballater for a much-needed break.

Mo has been incredibly stoic over her dental operation. So far, the implant surgery appears to have been very successful and the pain and swelling are gradually subsiding. Her lips are still a mess and she is having to monitor them to ensure that they are not infected. But she can now smile and be proud of her teeth which makes it all worthwhile.

9th June

Since my last entry Boris Johnson has survived a vote of confidence within the Tory party, although as many as 148 MPs supported the motion. Unsurprisingly, he is claiming this as a decisive victory and is openly unrepentant for his appalling behaviour. It remains to be seen how secure his position will remain if the Tories lose the forthcoming by-elections.

My mid-year appointment with the Parkinson's nurse was productive. She is much more focused and pro-active than her predecessor. In particular. she has given me clearer advice as to when to take my Co-careldopa and Ropinirole to ensure optimum effect. She is also adding a supplementary medication. However, she also seemed obsessed with the side-effects of Ropinirole – gambling and hyper-sexuality; needless to say, I was happy to reassure her!

The British economy and society seem to be encountering a perfect storm. Consumer confidence and domestic investment are at an historic low. The spiralling cost and supply constraints of raw materials are threatening to put many small and medium sized firms out of business. Some sectors, especially agriculture, are starved of labour due to Brexit and there is little sign that the much-vaunted trade agreements are in any way going to compensate for the fall in trade with the EU. It is forecast that in 2023 Britain's economy will have the lowest growth rate (0%) in the G20 except for Russia. Meanwhile, the unprecedented erosion of family incomes is leading to rising levels of poverty and the prospect of crippling industrial disputes, not least in the transport sector. As of today, the cost of filling the tank of an average size family car exceeds £100. The NHS continues to operate at a crisis level and faces a backlog in elective surgery lasting years as well as a pressing need to address the increasing health needs of those suffering from long-Covid. The devolved administrations are faring no better. The Scottish economy is performing poorly and Kate Forbes, the Cabinet Finance Secretary, is widely regarded in the media as 'economically illiterate'.

IndyRef2 is still very much on the agenda and the behaviour of Boris and his cronies merely reinforces the case of those seeking independence. If anything, Northern Ireland presents an even greater threat to the stability of British politics, the egregious handling of the Brexit Protocol serving to alienate the DUP and precipitate the suspension of Stormont. And all this even before the geopolitical repercussions and global economic effects of the war in Ukraine, are taken into account!

15th June

A bad day yesterday. I had a strange turn in the morning and Mo called an ambulance. However, it was clearly due to low blood pressure probably brought on partly by my medication. As a result, after consultation with my health practice, my medication has been modified. Fortunately, I did not have to go to hospital, but my blood pressure is going to be closely monitored prior to a visit to my GP. All our neighbours were hugely supportive.

The day was not improved by the fact that Nicola Sturgeon chose to formally launch the SNP's campaign for IndyRef2 even though recent polls do not indicate any certainty that another referendum would secure a win for the "Yes' vote, and despite the urgent need to give priority to any number of other issues facing the Scottish economy and society. Not the least of her worries should be the recent 'up-tick' in Covid infections in Scotland due to sub-variants of the Omicron virus. It is estimated that 1 in 40 of the Scottish population is now infected and another wave of the pandemic is anticipated in the autumn.

The Westminster Mad Hatter's Tea Party continues apace with the first forcible airlift to Rwanda of alleged 'illegal immigrants' being abandoned in the face of rulings by the European Court of Human Rights. All at a cost to the taxpayer of half a million pounds! Meanwhile, hundreds of migrants are still crossing the English Channel daily.

17th June

Unfortunately, we have not shared in the glorious weather and record temperatures enjoyed down South. It has been warm but not sunny. Concerning news on the pandemic front. It appears that the number of cases in the UK has risen by a factor of 43% in the last week; mainly sub-variants BA.4 and BA.5 of Omicron that are highly contagious and resistant to the existing vaccines.

Meanwhile, Boris is up to his usual antics. His second ethics advisor has resigned, appalled by the 'odious', duplicitous intentions of the Government in its handling of trade agreements. Boris's response is merely to consider abandoning the post entirely, leaving his administration free from any ethical constraints. Moreover, to avoid facing difficult questions at home he has cancelled important meetings with northern industrialists and buggered off to Ukraine where he can play the 'statesman' and be sure of a warm reception.

20th June

As of tomorrow, a nationwide rail strike threatens transport chaos. The Government's response is to sit on its hands rather than take a proactive role in advancing conciliation. Instead, it seeks to pass a highly provocative law sanctioning the use of non-union, 'agency' labour during industrial disputes, effectively undermining trade union rights and poisoning future industrial relations. Ominously, a range of other public sector unions (including nurses, teachers and lawyers) is lobbying their members in preparation for strike action.

The SNP's first public memorandum in preparation for IndyRef2 *(Independence in the Modern World: Wealthier, happier, fairer: Why not Scotland)* is devoid of any substantive or credible economic analysis. There is no mention in the document of currency, pensions, income and expenditure, our 22% deficit, trade, investment, oil and gas, or business. It remains wedded to the mantra that an independent Scotland could 'borrow its way to prosperity', an increasingly delusional view in a world in which interest rates are rising inexorably.

Today promised to be an ideal day for Innerleithen. Weather was warm with just a gentle breeze. Sadly, after we had gone about half a mile, Mo suddenly fell her full length, having probably pulled a ligament. With the aid of my cane she was able to limp back to the car and fortunately, although painfully, managed to drive home, her foot swelling all the while.

25th June

An eventful week. It transpires that Mo has broken a bone in her ankle and now has her foot encased in a boot for several weeks. Suddenly we are faced with a whole set of logistical problems given that Mo cannot drive. Fortunately, neighbours, friends and family are all rallying round to help and we can use online deliveries for the basic foodstuffs.

The good news is that the Tories lost the two by-elections in Wakefield and Tiverton and Honiton, the latter with a swing of nearly 30% to the Liberal Democrats. There are fresh calls for Boris to resign but he has taken himself off to Rwanda of all places and insists he will remain in post.

The bad news is the decision of the US Supreme Court to overrule Roe v Wade and the constitutional right of American women to secure an abortion. It is a hugely retrograde step and yet another example of Trump's invidious influence on

US politics and society, given that he deliberately appointed pro-life judges to the Supreme Court. Should he secure a second term of office the danger is that the 'Moral Right' will proceed to undermine other reproductive rights relating to contraception and sex education.

Covid news is also concerning. The number of cases is continuing to spiral and it is estimated that, as of today, 1 in 20 people in Scotland are infected. With the removal of all restrictions relating to distancing, testing, and shielding, policymakers have essentially reconciled themselves to Covid remaining for the foreseeable future on a par with the annual flu epidemics; something we have to learn to live with while relying on vaccines and new medications to keep the level of hospitalisations at a manageable level. However, a growing concern is the likely impact of the next flu epidemic in the autumn given the low level of immunity arising from two years of reduced social contact under various lockdowns.

27th June

The Sunday papers rightly expose the extent to which Brexit has damaged the British economy. Compared with the average performance of similar advanced economies, it is calculated that it has led to a 5% shortfall in UK GDP, equivalent to an annual loss of £120 billion. In investment the UK performance has been 13.7% lower with a similar shortfall in the trade in goods. In fact, the trade figures are the worst on historical record. Sadly, other preoccupations such as the pandemic and the war in Ukraine have conspired to distract the public and policymakers from the signal failure of Brexit to fulfil its false promises.

30ᵗʰ June

Nicola Sturgeon has now formally proposed that IndyRef2 be held in October 2023. She has written to Boris Johnson seeking to negotiate a Section 30 Order, which, as in 2014, would temporarily transfer power to hold a referendum from Westminster to Holyrood. Unsurprisingly, Johnson has not shifted from his previous view that 'this is not the time' for a fresh referendum. Accordingly, she is seeking the decision of the Supreme Court as to the legality of such a move should Boris continue to prove uncooperative. In the event that the Court rules that Holyrood does not have the power to hold it, Sturgeon has declared that the next general election will be a 'de facto referendum' with the SNP 'standing on a single issue of independence'. This is a high-risk strategy for Nicola given that recent polls have indicated a gradual, albeit slight, shift of public opinion against independence.

The poverty of talent in the Cabinet is daily evident. I suppose some of their names – 'useless Eustace'/'failing Grayling'/'loathsome Leadsom'/'Hunt the C....'/'handless Hancock'/'Dormant Mordaunt'- should give us a clue to their incompetence. Yet others have names that can at best be deemed ironic; witness James Cleverly, Priti Patel, and Lord Adonis!

1ˢᵗ July

The news from 'Pestminster' gets worse by the day. Following on the resignation of the Chief Whip after the loss of recent bye-elections, the Deputy Chief Whip (Pincher by name and evidently pincher by nature) has now had to resign after getting drunk and groping two men in a private member's club – no pun intended!

Meanwhile, there are increasingly ominous signs on the pandemic front. The Omicron variant BA.5 appears to be extremely infectious and there has been a new surge in the level of infection within the community. The number of people infected rose by a third in the last week and as many as 1 in 18 people in Scotland now have the virus, putting the NHS in many areas back into crisis mode with ambulances waiting hours to offload patients and many patients waiting hours, if not days, for a bed.

The malign influence of Trump lives on in three recent decisions by the US Supreme Court, to which, when in office, he deliberately nominated social conservatives: the withdrawal of the constitutional right of women to seek abortions, the extension of the constitutional right of citizens to carry arms both at home and in public, and the curtailment of the power of the Environmental Protection Agency to regulate greenhouse gas emissions from United States power plants. All point to the fact that the USA is fast becoming a graveyard of progressive ideals and aspirations.

7th July

Dramatic events on both the personal and political fronts. On 3rd July I had a nasty fall in the kitchen which has left me with a very sore back and muscle spasm. Following on from the fall I managed to slide off my bed and wedge myself up against my trolley. Because of my back injuries I could not get any traction to get up and had to use my emergency alarm to call out the 'fall team'. The episode has further eroded my walking and I just hope that I will be pain free soon so that I can be fit for my birthday celebrations. Meanwhile, Mo is contending with both her dental and ankle issues, along with the logistical problems now that she cannot drive.

On the political front, a sensational series of resignations from Tory Government and Party posts has culminated this morning in Boris Johnson reluctantly agreeing to step down as Prime Minister. Rishi Sunak and Sajid Javid led the revolt last weekend and by this morning there had been over sixty resignations. The sacking of Gove last night appears to have been decisive in sealing Johnson's fate. The situation is unprecedented with some departments having no ministerial representation. The debate has now focused on whether Boris can remain in post until a new Prime Minister is appointed or whether a caretaker Prime Minister should be appointed. If Boris stays, one is left wondering what damage he might wreak! As I write it is clear that he is determined to stay on. He is already appointing a new bunch of ministerial nonentities – James Cleverly for education (The third Minister of Education in three days!) - the irony of it all! Meanwhile, the Labour leaders are threatening to move a vote of confidence in the Government if Boris does not depart immediately.

11th July

My body is not in good shape. I still have severe discomfort in my lower back and left hand. Painkillers take the edge off the pain but the added stress on my body due to my freezing and festination creates further strain.

We are now being subjected to the unseemly sight of all Johnson's erstwhile sycophants bidding to be the next Prime Minister despite their collusion in his toxic antics in recent years. All the usual suspects have come out of the woodwork and appear to be vigorously briefing against each other. Political observers predict that it is likely to become the dirtiest leadership campaign in history. Typical is Dominic Cummings's evaluation of some of the early runners: 'At least three current candidates would be worse than Boris. At least one is more insane than Truss, clearly unfit to be anywhere near nuclear codes. At least one is a SPAD shagger'.

15th July

Yet another fall today leaving me stiff and bruised. Fortunately, after a convoluted process, we have managed to secure an x-ray appointment for Monday. Hopefully it will only reveal soft tissue damage enabling me to get some physiotherapy. It looks as though I shall be using my wheelchair earlier than I had anticipated.

17th July

I am still very stiff and bruised and lacking in traction with my left leg. However, the strains in my back and hand feel better. The infection levels of Omicron have once again risen by as much as a third in the last seven days and it is estimated that as many as one in sixteen of the Scottish population are currently infected. Another dear friend is the latest to test positive. To add to the crisis in the NHS we now have an amber alert for extreme heat with its associated health risks. Fortunately, by the time of my family do next weekend the temperature in Dalkeith will be a comfortable 18–20 degrees.

The campaign to select a new Tory leader has quickly deteriorated into a 'gong show' with a great deal of 'blue on blue' infighting. Thankfully, it looks as though Liz Truss will not make it through to the final round. Her performance so far, dressed in a hideous fauxThatcher outfit, has been woeful.

Anyone who claims on air that growing up she was a 'professional controversialist' deserves to be ridiculed.

19th July

80 today! Appropriately it is forecast to be the hottest day on record. Yesterday, I had an x-ray and CT scan on my left hip. Fortunately, no fracture showed up but apparently I have acute arthritis in my left hip. I just hope my present discomfort stems from muscle damage.

The behaviour of Johnson and his cronies in yesterday's no confidence debate was outrageous. The motion was deliberately staged to enable Boris to bow out without a word of contrition and made a mockery of parliament. The very people who had resigned from his Government were there baying in support of his grandiose claims to a place in history. Everything was geared to feed his narcissism, and the sad fact is that many people see this fatal flaw in his character as charisma! It will be interesting to see whether he remains in the Commons or indeed, accepts a Cabinet post. For sure, as with Trump in the USA, Boris is not done with trashing the democratic processes of governance.

26th July

My family birthday celebrations on the 23rd and 24th July went wonderfully well thanks to the enormous amount of planning and preparation by Mo, the invaluable help of Hilary and Martin, and the loving support of our neighbours; in particular, the inspired offer of a gazebo that enabled people to spread out into the garden. The weather was warm and dry, the food excellent and everyone was on good form. Mo made a lovely welcoming speech that acknowledged the efforts that people had made to travel to the party given the current transport chaos and the high incidence of Omicron. My brother, Colin, also said a few words, as did Andy who had flown over from Canada, before we downed our champagne. Thereafter, everyone chilled out and mingled way into the evening. The following day, they all turned up again to hoover up the remaining food and drink and it was a delight to have so much quality time with them all. The house now seems so quiet and empty.

Today I had some physiotherapy at home, and it is evident that I was very lucky not to have broken my hip given the amount of bruising I still have. The physiotherapist has given me some exercises to straighten and ease my left leg and advice on how to use my trolley without leaning on it.

2nd August

I had yet another fall this week. Fortunately, I did not really hurt myself, but the fact that I have fallen 4 times now in the last 2 months is a real worry. Online information indicates that falling is a very common aspect of stage 3 Parkinson's.

It appears that we are now reconciled to living with the pandemic. It is increasingly relegated to a minor slot in the media, with the spread of monkey pox and avian flu capturing the headlines. Certainly, it was noticeable that the likely spread of Omicron amongst the crowds attending and celebrating the women's European Cup Final and the Commonwealth Games elicited no comment in the press.

I have been reading Antony Bevor's book on the Russian Revolution and Civil War. An amazing feat of research but too much detail and too little contextual analysis. Unlike his brilliant study of Stalingrad this volume, in trying to capture the chaos and complexity of the civil war, made it almost impossible to see the wood for the trees; but I suppose in many ways the participants were similarly handicapped.

5th August

Last night we hosted a birthday party for twenty friends at Howies. It was hugely successful and amazingly we had a full turnout except for one friend who was very sadly trying to cope with the trauma of his computer and bank accounts having been scammed. Everyone was on good form, and it was especially lovely to see two old friends with whom I have kept in close contact now for over 50 years. Mo made a very funny impromptu speech. Thanks to her efforts it all went off seamlessly, and Gayle's selfless offer to transport us to and from the event hugely added to the enjoyment of the evening.

However, a call this morning informing us that my brother has been hospitalised with severe bladder and prostate problems is very worrying and we await updates.

On the political front, the latest forecasts by the Bank of England are dire. In order to try and curb inflation (now predicted to peak at over 13%, the highest level for 42 years) the Bank has raised Bank Rate by 0.5 % with further rises anticipated in the autumn. Moreover, the Bank has confirmed its previous warnings that we are entering the longest recession since the financial crisis of 2007–08. Ofgem is now predicting that, by the New Year, the yearly energy bill for the average household may reach at least £3,800!

The infection levels for Omicron appear to be trending slightly downward, although the news that some 5,700 people in Scotland are still suffering from the side effects of long Covid after 12 months suggests that the pandemic may be taking its toll on the nation's health for years to come.

10th August

The estimated fuel bill for the typical household in 2023 has now risen to over £4200!! and the issue of fuel poverty has come to dominate the Tory leadership campaign. Unless some substantive rescue policy is devised the impact on the level of fuel poverty this coming winter will be catastrophic.

Colin seems to be making a slow recovery in hospital. He was clearly very traumatised by the episode and is still telling a bizarre tale of being left in a trolley on the top floor of the hospital within inches of a forty-foot drop. My niece had warned me that he was clearly hallucinating when he went into hospital. He still has a catheter in and needs assistance to walk any distance, and it is difficult to assess how serious his condition really is. We suspect that dehydration and a urine infection were the initial causes of his distress, but we also have concerns about his cognitive health.

11th August

This week has seen record temperatures with heat alerts across much of the country. Today it is 30 degrees in Edinburgh and the garden is looking thoroughly parched. An official drought has been declared in many areas of England. Just one more challenge to add to the litany of problems facing our policy makers.

The news from Suffolk is mixed. On the one hand, Colin's condition is no longer viewed as serious. On the other, we are clearly not alone in detecting some signs of confusion and memory loss.

The Omicron pandemic continues to be marginalised in the media and overshadowed by the energy and cost of living crises. However, the increasing incidence of monkey pox and the re-emergence of polio in the UK years after it was considered to be eradicated, should keep the virologists and epidemiologists on their toes!

26th August

An eventful fortnight. The journey up to Ballater was scenically stunning but there then followed two days of rain. As it turned out, the lodge was not accessible as it had no shower and no grab rails. In future, we need to be far more specific in listing our requirements. On the third day, we managed to have a two-hour run in the scooter, following a well-surfaced path from Ballater station. However, I felt utterly exhausted and under par for the rest of the day. By the evening, after Hilary and Martin had set off home, I was running a temperature and becoming incontinent and increasingly unwell. There followed nine hours of waiting for an ambulance with no support from the hotel. Fortunately, the local GP was able to book me straight into a ward bed in Aberdeen Royal Infirmary where I gradually recovered over the next week. The situation was hugely stressful, as Mo did not feel confident to drive home without support should I take ill en route. Various plans were devised but for a variety of reasons they all unravelled. Eventually, I recovered sufficiently to enable Mo to drive me home. A great deal of expense with little respite!

Back to the perfect storm of rising inflation, unprecedented falls in real earnings and looming catastrophic rises in fuel costs. Today the energy price cap for October has risen by a further 80% with the annual fuel bill for the average household now estimated at over £3,500, with further significant rises anticipated.

Meanwhile, Boris is on his third holiday and policymaking is in limbo while a new Tory leader and Cabinet emerges. Strikes are breaking out across all sectors in protest at the erosion of living standards, even involving criminal barristers. The most visible effects can be seen in the Scottish cities, where the cessation of bin collection is causing mountains of rubbish to build up and a fresh plague of rats to emerge. Hopefully, this is not a metaphor for the breakdown of civil society in the months to come! The Government is faced with what appears to be an impossible dilemma. The rise in living costs will inevitably erode disposable incomes and suppress domestic consumption that in turn will help drag the economy into a period of recession. At the same time, to control rising inflation, interest rates need to rise thus imposing an additional burden on house owners and other borrowers. Meanwhile, employers' associations are predicting that the impact of spiralling energy costs on the leisure industry, and more generally on small and medium-sized businesses, will lead to widespread redundancies and closures.

1st September

Everything seems dysfunctional. My health is suspect; my mobility is worse, and I have lost confidence in accessing the garden and the feeders. My sleep pattern is very erratic and must I suspect take its toll on my energy levels and periods of tremor and agitation. In addition, I have been diagnosed with another UTI that is known to affect cohesion and mobility in the elderly. My only contribution over the last week has been to core the first windfall of apples. The positives have been the on-line sessions from the Edinburgh International Book Festival – Michael Ignatieff, Ian Rankin, Liz Lochhead, and Antony Bevor.

Sadly, Colin is still in hospital following his stroke. They are awaiting some sort of care package that will enable Ann to cope with him at home, especially with respect to showering. The damage to his eyesight is going to make it difficult for him to navigate their house. At the moment a good deal of what he says makes no sense, but they hope this will improve as his brain recovers.

The political news is really depressing with the very real prospect of Liz Truss becoming Prime Minister! She is profoundly ignorant of economic issues and has no talent for diplomacy. It is not beyond the realms of possibility that she will be incapable of coping with the cost of living and energy crises, thus precipitating an early election at which Boris will re-emerge as Tory leader.

International news is also distressing. Over 10% of Pakistan is under flood water and suffering a major disaster with over 30 million people displaced and much of the infrastructure destroyed. Meanwhile, drought and famine are again visiting the Horn of Africa. In Western Europe, Putin has effectively weaponised the supply of gas and successfully created an ongoing fuel crisis with its associated impact on inflation, living standards and industrial relations. Ukrainian forces appear to be gradually developing a counter-offensive in Kherson. However, there is continuing concern that the fighting may endanger the nuclear plant at Zaporizhzhia and trigger a nuclear disaster. News from the East is equally threatening, with China playing military brinkmanship over Taiwan and compelling evidence of genocide against the Uyghurs and other Muslim minority groups in Xinjiang.

And where in all this is the pandemic? It has curiously slipped off the headlines despite the fact that the NHS remains overstretched, and some virologists are predicting a major Covid/flu epidemic by October. While deaths and hospital admissions in Scotland involving Covid are now trending downwards, the Scottish administration has still not addressed the legacy of long

Covid and there is a strong sense that, in terms of the pandemic, we are experiencing a brief calm before the storm.

5th September

Liz Truss is to be the new Prime Minister!! And the Mad Hatter's Tea Party enters a new chapter. Matthew Syed in the *Sunday Times* aptly summed up the protracted campaign for the Tory leadership as 'ship hands on the titanic arguing to rearrange the deckchairs'.

10th September

Queen Elizabeth II died on 8th September at the age of 96, to be succeeded by Charles III. To my surprise I found that I felt quite emotional at her passing. Amidst all the hype, hypocrisy, and hubris of recent political events, she remained a force for stability and selflessness. It remains to be seen if Charles can steer the monarchy with equal finesse in years to come.

12th September

As I feared, the ceremonial proceedings surrounding the monarchy have totally overshadowed other issues that require urgent attention. We have already suffered weeks of inaction due to the change of Tory leadership, and we can ill-afford further delay in addressing the fuel and cost of living crises, as well as the ongoing crisis in the NHS.

Better news from Ukraine where Russian troops have suffered a significant defeat and appear to be retreating from some strategic towns in the occupied territories. My only fear is that the more Putin is humiliated by military setbacks the more likely it is that he will deploy nuclear weaponry or compromise the safety of the reactor at Zaporizhzhia.

Sad news from Suffolk. Colin is clearly struggling. I am swithering as to whether I should travel south to see him in case the worst happens. It is a difficult call. The prospect of the demise of yet another constant in my life is distressing.

21st September

Better news of Colin. His condition seems to have stabilised, and I was able to have a fairly cogent phone call with him at the weekend. This week has been dominated by the State funeral of Elizabeth 11. I found some of the proceedings quite emotional, albeit I find the very concept of 'monarchy' repellent and much of the royal saga socially repugnant.

Meanwhile, Liz Truss is strutting her stuff like a teenager on speed! Her first action on entering office was to dismiss the Permanent Secretary to the Treasury. Unbelievably, she has also signed off on proposals to remove the present cap on bankers' bonuses! She talks in vacuous sound bites about promoting growth in a more technically advanced economy but signally fails to acknowledge that it is the immediate prospect of widespread fuel and food poverty that needs addressing. Her most recent warning that she will have to take some unpopular decisions bodes ill for the mass of the population. If it all goes pear-shaped the Tory backbenches, ever mindful of their electoral fortunes, will soon disown her.

Today, Putin raised the odds in the war in Ukraine by holding referenda in some of the occupied territories on whether they wish to reintegrate with Russia. He warns that should they so wish, any subsequent support from NATO to Ukrainian forces will be seen as a direct attack on Russia, at which point all defence weapons, including nuclear weapons, will be deployed. The prospect of a nuclear disaster was also heightened by the news that a rocket had narrowly missed the nuclear reactor at Zaporizhzhia.

23rd September

The Government has taken a huge gamble with a mini budget that contains tax cuts to the tune of 45 billion pounds, on a scale only previously seen in the ill-fated Barber budget of 1972. Liz Truss is obsessed with economic growth and openly claims that the issue of 'redistribution' is less important than stimulating the economy to the benefit of all. So much for 'social levelling'! A whole range of proposed tax cuts is weighted in favour of the wealthiest in society. In addition, it is proposed to cancel the current cap on banker's bonuses. We have now a fundamental conflict between the Bank of England, whose aim is to raise interest rates in an effort to curb the level of inflation, and the Chancellor of the Exchequer, Kwasi Kwarteng, who, in accordance with Liz Truss's naïve economic philosophy, seeks to stimulate greater economic activity regardless of its inflationary repercussions. Already, the pound has further weakened against the dollar and the Euro, and there has been a predictable fall on the stock markets. It is evident that many Tory MPs are very unhappy with the scale and 'optics' of these proposals. Indeed, one backbencher was heard to remark that, in effect, this was 'the UK filing for bankruptcy'.

28th September

Unsurprisingly, Kwasi's mini budget (now dubbed the 'Kamikaze' budget) with its perverse adherence to tax cuts, while at the same time accruing massive debt, has spooked the money markets. There has been an immediate and significant fall in the value of sterling and in the FTSE index. More seriously, the bond market has been severely affected which will increase the size of the national debt even further and put more pressure on bank and mortgage rates. In an unprecedented intervention today, the IMF has warned that the current strategy of the Treasury is unsustainable; a view shared by many economists and the Bank of England.

To add to our woes, public health experts are warning of a 'Twindemic' this winter of flu and Coronavirus. I shall be mightily relieved when we get our vaccinations next week.

29th September

Due to the crass mismanagement of the economy by Truss and Kwarteng the Treasury was yesterday compelled to pump huge sums of money into the economy to protect pension funds against the rise in the cost of borrowing on the bond market. And just at a time when the Bank of England is struggling to use higher interest rates to curb inflation. There is a desperate need for the Government to get control of the situation as there is a real fear that this strategy of unfunded tax cuts will ruin confidence in Britain in the money markets and trigger a complete melt down. This grief is so needlessly self-inflicted. Had the former experienced Permanent Secretary to the Treasury not been unceremoniously discarded and had Kwarteng's mini budget been submitted to the Office of Budget Responsibility in line with normal practice, the folly of pursuing a policy that spooked the money and mortgage markets could have been avoided. I think Liz Truss's tenure in office is likely to be a very brief one unless the markets settle down in the next few days.

2nd October

It transpires that taxpayers may be left with an estimated bill of £34 billion pounds to compensate the Bank of England for losses it has incurred buying billions of pounds of government bonds to avoid a crisis in the pension funds industry. It is reported that Liz Truss is called 'Dagger' by her civil servants as it is short for Dagenham which is only two stops short of Barking! Her political future hangs on a thread.

9th October

The Tory conference was predictably a car crash with Truss desperately reiterating her 'trickle down' philosophy; promising the earth without any serious analysis and critical disregard for the debt implications and for the collateral damage that she had already inflicted on the mortgage and bond markets. When Parliament reconvenes, we are in for some lively debate, not least because she clearly lacks the backing of many in her own party.

Thankfully, we have now had our flu and Omicron vaccinations. It is a great relief as there is growing evidence of a new wave of the pandemic arriving in the UK affecting older people in particular, and the health and care services are already fully stretched with patients waiting hours for medical attention.

11th October

A depressing week on a number of fronts. Our dear friends have been in a bad road accident and recovering from various bruises and strains, and emotional trauma. News from Suffolk is not good. Colin clearly needs constant back-up. His eyesight is still impaired, and his memory loss is all too apparent.

On the political front, the Government's strategy continues to harbour a basic tension between monetary and fiscal objectives. A range of U turns has been adopted to reassure the financial markets, but, as of today, the Bank of England is still warning that it may have to intervene in order to head off a complete collapse in confidence in the viability of the Tory budget. The sad fact is that Kwarteng has still to convince most economic observers that his tax proposals are adequately funded without having to introduce yet another period of cuts. A lot will depend on the forthcoming, albeit scandalously delayed, report of the Office of Budget Responsibility, assuming the financial system will not by then have gone into melt down.

The long-term impact of Covid and its related restrictions on the nation's cultural life is increasingly evident. The Edinburgh Filmhouse has this week gone into administration and the National Galleries are predicting severely reduced opening hours.

15th October

It is difficult to keep up with the 'Westminster gong show'. Yesterday, Liz Truss had the temerity to sack her Chancellor (the fourth in three months) but to remain in post herself. She held a disastrous press conference where she simply repeated ad nauseam her mantra about 'growth' and displayed not one iota of shame for the damage that has been done to the money and bond markets and to Britain's financial rating, not to mention the adverse effects on the level of inflation and mortgage rates. Significantly, rather than calming the markets, her press conference created even more instability and the value of the pound fell back. In Kwarteng's place, she has appointed Jeremy Hunt, notwithstanding his previous inept handling of health policy over many years.

As I write, the pressure on Truss to resign is steadily mounting. Many leading backbench Tories are of the opinion that she has 'trashed' the reputation of the Party for fiscal discipline and competence and that she cannot be allowed to lead it into the next election. However, how a further change in the premiership could be affected without creating further distraction from the immediate issues of fuel, food, and housing poverty, as well as the crisis in the health and care systems, is problematic. One possible option would be to make Hunt Prime Minister and bring back Rishi Sunak as Chancellor. Whatever transpires, at the very least Truss must surely go! Interestingly, there is a widespread conviction in much of the media that after this complete unravelling of governance the Tories are doomed to take a heavy defeat at any general election.

21st October

So, the 'gong show' continues. Liz Truss resigned yesterday afternoon without a sliver of contrition or self-deprecation and without any apology for screwing up the economy and wrecking Britain's financial reputation. The shortest tenure of the premiership in British political history. Cynics that predicted that she would not outlast the shelf-life of a supermarket lettuce have been duly vindicated! Those who supported her bid for the post are equally culpable. And now we are faced with the prospect of Boris resubmitting himself for the role. The Tories are arguing that he is the only person with a democratic mandate (from the last general election) and they see him as their only chance of avoiding wipe-out in any future election. The fact that he was so recently ejected from Office as an inveterate liar has been conveniently forgotten in their desperate attempts to save their seats. Unfortunately, there are many in the Tory Party, both in Parliament and the constituencies, who would be happy to see his return. It is a depressing thought that Parliament could once again be exposed to his vacuous, divisive showmanship at a time when the policy community needs mature, considered leadership. What an unholy mess!

28th October

We now have Rishi Sunak as PM and Hunt remaining as Chancellor of the Exchequer. It is difficult to comprehend just what Tory policy is now given that Truss's growth strategy has been systematically rejected. To all intents and purposes, we are likely to endure yet another period of 'austerity' to appease the money markets.

I feel my Parkinson's has entered another plateau. My balance is bad, but the new patches have had a dramatic effect in reducing my dribbling. If anything, my tremor is better. We used the scooter at Flotterstone earlier this week and it added another venue that worked for us.

3rd November

It is difficult to capture all the dismal news on so many fronts. The Bank of England is predicting the longest recession since records began in the 1920s. Sunak is full of foreboding, and it is clear we are in for another severe bout of austerity with cuts to many of the services that are already in crisis, not excluding education and health. Major projects such as the building of a new nuclear plant and the modernisation of the northern rail system are being reviewed. The 'triple lock' on pensions also looks vulnerable. The sheer size of the savings to be made, only exacerbated by the Truss/Kwarteng debacle, means that few areas of activity will be immune. Meanwhile, the fuel crisis is already putting many firms and outlets out of business and driving thousands of families into fuel as well as food poverty. The international situation provides little solace. The mid-term elections in the USA threaten a replay of the violence that accompanied Biden's appointment as President with Trump again on the rampage. In Ukraine, the Ukrainians are making slow progress in driving the Russian army out, but most worryingly the safety of the nuclear plant at Zaporizhzhia has been compromised by shelling.

Colin is 85 today. Thankfully, apart from his eyesight he seems to be recovering well, although there are significant blanks in his memory. He professed no knowledge of our disastrous trip to Ballater. We are hoping to arrange a Zoom tomorrow so at least we can have visual contact with them all.

11th November

The birthday Zoom was a great success. It was lovely to see all the family and they were obviously enjoying our champagne present. A mixed week. I had a very enjoyable visit to Vane Farm despite the very blustery weather. The stars of the visit were a little egret and a cluster of pintails. I am gradually learning how to keep warm and strategies for getting the most out of our visits. A valium before we set out enables me to be more relaxed.

I have been pushing on with a fair amount of ancestry work. As I move into the 18th century, the absence of a census makes life difficult. Some work was done by dad with the help of a professional genealogist, but I need to dig further into the Scottish records. I also managed to complete a book review which was an enjoyable intellectual exercise.

Healthwise, a mixed week. The patches continue to alleviate my dribbling and my new tablet, designed to reinforce the Co-careldopa, appears to be reducing my tremor, although it also produces some weird dreams. I have also decided to be more proactive in arranging for the routine checks for dental and visual health that I always had before the pandemic. Most of the medical and dental services appear to have retreated from sight unless they are challenged.

The political mood remains febrile. We are clearly entering yet another period of 'austerity' with 'Hunt the C...' promising 'eye-watering' measures that will inevitably add to the unrest already triggered by the escalation in the cost of living. In addition to a succession of rail stoppages, strikes are impending in the health and education services. We are now officially entering what is predicted to be the longest recession in modern British history with manufacturing growth well below pre-pandemic levels. Hell mend the mindless idiots who supported Brexit!

18th November

Yesterday, Hunt presented his emergency budget statement in a desperate attempt to regain the confidence of the money markets. Today's *Scotsman* rightly styles it the 'Nightmare before Christmas'. Underlying the bland promises of the Government are some stark realities. The self-indulgent ego trip of Truss is said to have wiped '£30 billion off the public purse'. We are now at the start of a protracted recession. Inflation is now running at 11.1% and is predicted to remain at around 7% in 2023, wiping out the previous eight years of economic growth. In the coming months there will be the biggest decline in real household incomes since the early 1950s. Moreover, not only are we left with the highest tax burden since the Second World War but the annual repayment of interest on the national debt is also predicted to rise to over 100 billion pounds, greater than the cost of any public service, bar the NHS. Amidst all this neither party is prepared to acknowledge the additional damage inflicted on our trade and industry by Brexit!

On the Parkinson's front, I am disgusted at the casual way my appointment with my consultant has simply been deferred, without explanation, for another six months. Fortunately, I have felt more stable in the last few weeks. The patches have certainly reduced my incessant dribbling and the Entacapone seems to have reduced my tremor. I just need to be aware of the danger of low blood pressure first thing in the morning and to allow time for my cornucopia of pills to process. I was greatly moved by an invitation to the Parentline Christmas party. It will be lovely to see all the staff and volunteers again. My phone befriending is going well and there is a possibility of my taking on a second client in the near future.

25th November

A mixture of a week. Some positives. My AAA scan indicated that the aneurism was virtually the same as two years ago and the technician saw no reason for any more appointments. This afternoon we go for our first optician's appointment in two years. Hopefully I will escape with just a change of lenses and not yet needing treatment for cataracts. *[In fact, no change in lenses was required and although there are the predictable traces of age-related cataracts, my condition was way away from needing any referral]* Then, tomorrow we pack for a short break at Crieff Hydro which hopefully will prove more enjoyable than our Ballater fiasco.

I am still sticking to my exercise and guitar routines and focusing on my leg strength by using my exercise bike in the conservatory. There is a pre-Christmas lethargy and I find it difficult to enthuse about the festive season. It is for many people a sad time of regrets and loss and there is a real feeling of vulnerability now the NHS is in such a parlous state. This is not a time to be ill or suffer injuries and I am constantly backing out of tasks through fear of falling, and this merely reinforces my lack of confidence.

The courts have dealt a body blow to Sturgeon's ambitions to hold a referendum on Scottish independence next year, provoking a predictable array of protest meetings from SNP supporters. Instead, Nicola proposes that the next general election should be regarded as constituting a proxy referendum.

Ukraine presents a sorry picture. The Ukrainians have succeeded in frustrating Putin's original aims but are resigned to a prolonged war. How long NATO can afford to be funding them if hostilities continue into 2023 is a moot point, especially when there are so many calls on government funding at home. Meanwhile, Putin is devastating the infrastructure of Ukraine by targeting its water and energy utilities and leaving the population to freeze and starve as the winter sets in.

Colin is very much in my thoughts. I cannot imagine a world without my brother. We are so different in manner and ideology, but he has always been there for me and never resented my early opportunities of an uninterrupted education and freedom from National Service and has always been the most hospitable of hosts, apart from his obsession with saving money on heating!

28th November

Our weekend break to Crieff was blessed with some beautiful views and clear sunny weather. Due to abnormal weather patterns the trees still retained a legacy of autumnal colours, and the mountains were spectacular – Perthshire at its very best. The Hydro, as always, was extremely friendly and supportive and the Indian food in the restaurant, now headed by a Michelin Star chef, was outstanding. However, what struck me most about the hotel was the absence of any reference to the pandemic. We are truly learning to live with it and to normalise the infection.

Reading the *Sunday Times* has left me with an apocalyptic view of the world with a perfect storm approaching. Looking abroad, there is the likelihood of the war in Ukraine at best ending in a brokered peace settlement, with the world's geopolitics fundamentally fractured and reset, and with the inevitable collateral damage to the world's energy and food supply routes. There is also the continuing possibility of a nuclear accident at Zaporizhzhia. In addition, there is the strong possibility of Trump regaining the Presidency and the continuing threat of another pandemic. Meanwhile, at home, there is the prospect of strike action engulfing the country with an associated rise in civil unrest and increasingly violent social conflict engendered by the rise in the cost of living, the battle over IndyRef2, and the total breakdown in health and care services. Despite the 'gong show' surrounding the premierships of May, Johnson, and Truss there is no indication that the Tories are going to adopt a more inclusive, distributive approach to politics nor to hold accountable those ministers and officials who presided over the defrauding of British taxpayers during the pandemic.

9th December

Yesterday we received our first snowfall and the temperature has suddenly dropped. Winter is definitely announcing its arrival, despite several of the garden roses still in flower. Today we went to Restoration Yard for lunch. It went well logistically especially as I am still able to use the walker some distance. Delightful to see good friends for some quality time. Apart from Mo's reheated microwave curry, the food was good. It was surreal to be eating normally again in a restaurant with no masks and an atmosphere of normality.

The state of the country continues to depress. There are so many unions calling for strike action that we are virtually facing a 'General Strike' over the Christmas and New Year period. Added to my general sense of doom is the sudden announcement of the 'deprecation of Microsoft basic authentication' that effectively means I no longer have connection between my apple mail app. and the University e-mail system and must access my emails via MyEd. So, sadly it looks as though I finally will have to reconcile myself to buying a new computer in the New Year.

Another fall this week in the bedroom. Fortunately, I was able to use my mobile phone to alert Mo and I was able to get up safely without any damage, other than to my physical confidence.

14th December

So far, no more snow but a hard frost has made going out very risky. Our annual book group Christmas get together was very successful, but we are all ageing and much of the conversation was very much an 'organ recital'.

The tree looks great and Mo has, as usual, decorated it tastefully. The crackers I bought were a great disappointment and hugely over-priced. I was not impressed with my dental treatment. The dentist only gave my teeth a cursory glance and there was no real exploration of how my teeth were feeling. He recommended a repair filling, but it will cost £276! In addition, he recommended three-monthly hygiene appointments, but once again it will incur considerable expenditure. Somehow the former NHS tariff, for which we registered, seems to have been buried by the Covid procedures. It certainly feels that even routine treatment has been effectively privatised.

We are now experiencing an 'advent calendar' of industrial disputes with a range of unions opting for strike action over the festive season. The railways are effectively paralysed until mid-January, the postal service is subject to stoppages and there is still the prospect of the nursing profession striking in England and Wales. There is a real feeling that Brexit and the egregious behaviour of the Tory Government has left British society fractured and its economy severely weakened.

However, taking the long view, perhaps the most significant news yesterday was the announcement that scientists in America had successfully produced nuclear fusion that in the future could provide limitless energy with minimal impact on the environment.

16th December

Forecast of snow has meant the cancellation of most of our plans but, given that Mo is feeling under par, it may be a blessing. Two nights ago I went on my own to the Parentline Christmas party; the first time I have ventured forth on my own since March 2020! All went well and people were wonderfully supportive and welcoming. It feels like a real boost to my self-esteem and hopefully I can be more proactive in getting out to the cinema and theatre.

Putin is doing his best to 'weaponise' energy supplies and to leave Ukrainians freezing to death by systematically targeting their power generation facilities with drones. There must surely come a time when NATO either feels compelled to resort to direct force or to put pressure on Zelensky to settle for a compromise peace.

Straws in the wind: In England and Wales hospital admissions are now more related to the flu virus rather than the Coronavirus pandemic. I suspect there are more medical challenges to come before the winter is over.

22nd December

Time to begin to reflect on another year. The highpoints were my 80th parties that were hugely enjoyable. The low points revolved around health issues: Mo's dental work and broken ankle and my various falls and hospitalisation in Aberdeen. But we did manage to stay safe from the pandemic and have gradually come to terms with the fact that it is going to be part of our lives in years to come. My Parkinson's proceeds to dominate my life but I am still mentally positive and doing all I can to slow the course of degeneration. Compared with this time last year I am certainly more unbalanced and subject to festination, but my voice is still okay, as is my appetite. Recent changes in my medication have reduced my tremors and dribbling, although sadly they cannot affect my mobility. It is walking that I miss most. As before, I have had minimal support from the NHS. I have not seen my consultant for three years; only a few cursory phone reviews, and my current appointment has been deferred to May 2023 without any explanation. In many ways it has made little difference to my condition as there is still no cure for Parkinson's and consultations had a limited value, but it is just another example of the pitiful state of the NHS.

British politics is sick. We are being led by a bunch of amoral, second-rate nonentities whose main agenda appears to be their own self-aggrandisement. The Truss debacle was hugely entertaining but laid bare the moral and intellectual bankruptcy of the Tory Government. The 'advent calendar' of industrial disputes, (both active and forthcoming) continues to paralyse the country and ruin any travel plans over the festive season. It is a vicious circle. The unions are desperate to secure for their members a settlement that both redresses the fall in real incomes during the period of austerity and that compensates for the current inflation of living costs. Meanwhile, the Treasury is determined to avoid the further inflation that would inevitably follow, especially in the absence of any rise in labour productivity.

A chilling final Reith Lecture on the geopolitical situation arising out of the invasion of Ukraine. The speaker was at pains to emphasise that we are now effectively in a Third World War, and we need to respond appropriately. Equally chilling is the failure of the British Government to take immediate action to impose border controls and restrictions on Chinese arrivals in line with several other countries. Clearly the sudden withdrawal of lockdown in China has created a massive rise in the incidence of Covid-19 and its variants along with associated deaths. There must be a strong probability that within this maelstrom a new variant will emerge that is resistant to current vaccines. It seems inexcusable that our leaders have not introduced appropriate measures to prevent its spread to the UK.

PART IV

Exiting the Pandemic 2023

2ⁿᵈ January

We saw the New Year in with our neighbours. The usual 'organ recital' followed by lengthy discussion of the Gender Recognition Reform Bill.

My previous entry for once perhaps does the policy community an injustice. On this occasion, the Government has taken swift action to police arrivals from China, despite the view of several leading epidemiologists that imposing additional restrictions on travellers has little effect on the spread of the Coronavirus and that any new variant would already be circulating in the UK. The Government rightly distrusts the pandemic information coming out of China and wants, at all costs, to avoid another lockdown.

Colin seems to be gradually improving and I was able to have a clear and cogent telephone conversation with him yesterday. His sight and mobility have clearly been affected and he often struggles to remember names and events, but he sounded far less confused and in good spirits.

Grim news from the Royal College of Emergency Medicine that the crisis in A&E departments due to staff and bed shortages was estimated to be leading to hundreds of excess deaths.

5ᵗʰ January

Disturbing news that a new Coronavirus variant, xbb1.5, is sweeping the USA. It is said to be highly infectious, and we do not know how far our existing vaccines will cope with it. Similarly, the outcome of the sudden Chinese withdrawal of pandemic restrictions is yet to be identified.

The melt down of the NHS worsens daily, with critically ill patients waiting hours, if not days, before being discharged from ambulances, and then being treated on trollies and even in cupboards due to an acute shortage of beds. The dental services are little better with NHS-funded work limited to the bare minimum. The rest is defined as private work and is hugely expensive. For example, today I had two fillings costing me £558! In many areas the dental service is now effectively privatised and it seems unlikely that we will ever return to the pre-pandemic world. There is a strong suspicion that the Government will use the current crisis as an excuse to privatise the whole care system.

11th January

More and more horror stories from those working on the front line in the NHS, and another nursing strike scheduled later this week. The flu seems to have been particularly dangerous in the elderly, especially when it is part of a lethal cocktail of flu, Coronavirus and strep A infections. I feel flat and unfulfilled as I near the end of my ancestry work.

The weather doesn't help; grey, dreich and uninviting. Having reached 80 I am struggling to find new targets that will sustain me. The prospect of having to acquire a new computer and to become conversant with all the newer apps depresses me, but sadly the time has come for me to replace my MacBook Pro and take on board the new world of the 21st Century.

18th January

I have been feeling under par the last few days with some episodes in the morning of feeling slightly nauseous and faint. I am pretty sure it is due to low blood pressure, possibly brought on by the Entacapone medication. Something (I suspect the new thicker curtains in my bedroom) has had a dramatic effect on my sleeping pattern and I am struggling to get up before 8am which goes against my ingrained work ethic.

At the end of last week we went to the Brunton Theatre to check out accessibility for forthcoming film presentations of National Theatre plays. Everyone was very supportive. In fact, my main worry is not access but how far my bladder will behave.

There is very little activity on the feeders. I find this surprising given that we are now in a cold spell with a covering of snow. I must content myself with watching Winterwatch on TV. Undoubtedly there would be rich viewing at Vane Farm but I would be frozen stiff on the scooter, even if the paths were manageable.

The 'apocalyptic' stories from the NHS continue unabated. Even patients with suspected strokes or heart attacks are waiting many hours, sometimes days, before receiving treatment on the hospital wards. Statistics from National Health Scotland reveal that last week less than 60% of attendances at A&E were seen within four hours, as compared with the official target of 90%. Meanwhile, elective surgery is often delayed for months, and in many cases, years. The rail service remains dire with on-going strikes and cancellations rendering any sort of travel hazardous and unpredictable.

The political scene remains fractious. Sturgeon has condemned the Tory Government for blocking the Gender Recognition Reform Bill passed by Holyrood, viewing it as a denial of Scotland's constitutional rights. In fact, this is one issue where we agree with Whitehall. The Bill would compromise the safety of women and serve to endorse the questionable interference with the normal processes of adolescent socio-sexual development. Meanwhile, there are clear signs of discontent within the SNP with growing pressure on Sturgeon to deliver Scottish Independence sooner rather the later. Blackford's displacement from the leadership of the SNP at Westminster is, I suspect, an early indication of more radical changes to come within the SNP.

21 January

Yesterday, we ventured forth to the cinema for the first time since the start of the pandemic to see Olivia Colman in *Empire of Light*; a very moving film brilliantly acted. The logistics worked well and I was able to manage with just my walker, and with the blue badge parking presented no problem. Hopefully, this may be the start of a more adventurous life. Next week we are booked to see *The Crucible* at the Brunton Theatre. It will be good to establish whether my walker will be sufficient. My intuition is that the scooter could be more trouble than it's worth. I have stopped taking the Entacapone and feel much less light-headed and faint in the morning.

The newspapers are dominated by the seemingly endless crisis within the NHS. There is increasing evidence that the previous regime of lockdown and self-distancing has left the population with little resistance to flu and the Strep A virus and that, in addition, long Covid will present a formidable challenge for months, if not years, to come. Morale within the NHS appears to be at rock bottom and the current strike action by nurses reflects how desperate the situation has become.

Meanwhile, the more contentious the issue of gender recognition has become, the more thankful I am no longer to be teaching a course on sexuality. In the current climate I would not have lasted five minutes. As Lord Coe rightly observed 'Sex always trumps Gender' and to equate what is a biologically given with what is socially constructed is nonsensical.

26th January

British governance appears to be irretrievably corrupted by rich Tory ministers who appear to believe that the tax laws are there to be broken and that 'conflict of interest' is not a valid reason for declining office. As a result, major issues relating to the NHS, inflation, immigration, gender recognition and industrial relations are starved of parliamentary time in favour of endless, rebarbative debate over the probity of ministers.

Midlothian's proposed cuts to meet a growing deficit in future years are hugely depressing. They anticipate the removal of all library staff and a drastic reduction in funding for voluntary services, along with a withdrawal of support for disability provisions such as Handicabs.

A big test tonight as we are due to attend the Brunton Theatre to watch a live, filmed version of *The Crucible* by the National Theatre. It will be interesting to see whether I can manage just with the walker.

27th January

Using the walker proved successful and the Brunton proved very accessible and supportive with adequate toilet facilities. The play was superb and totally compelling. Along with our recent visit to the cinema, the evening was very empowering and hopefully will encourage me to be more outgoing.

28th January

The papers make for a depressing read with an endless litany of sleaze and self-inflicted crises. It is difficult to capture them all but undoubtedly Brexit and the Truss debacle have dragged us back into yet another decade of 'austerity'. It is estimated that last week some 6,000 Scottish patients had to wait for over a day to receive treatment in A&E. To add to our slough of despond, Flybe has today gone into liquidation.

Possible sighting of redpoll on the beach at Longniddry Bents and a group of long-tailed tits on my garden feeders.

29th January

We have now watched three excellent films that may win an Oscar; The *Empire of Light* (at the cinema), *All Quiet on the Western Front* (home screening) and *The Banshees of Inisherin* (home screening). Indeed, we have watched more films and National Theatre productions in the last week than over the last three years. Last night we watched the National Theatre production of *Prima Facie*, a compelling solo performance by Jodie Corner examining the relationship of the law and legal system to sexual offences and the nature of consent.

My blood pressure readings are curiously mixed. Perfectly normal in the morning but unacceptably high by mid-afternoon. It will be interesting to see how the practice nurse receives them.

2nd February

Two medical appointments this week. I had a very supportive meeting with the practice nurse who took bloods. After some discussion, I decided to include the PSA test, despite its limitations. The nurse was concerned at my loss of weight and low BMI, and this is something I need to address. She did not think my blood pressure readings were a cause for concern. I found the session with the Parkinson's nurse less helpful. For some reason, probably because I was feeling off-colour, I was really agitated and my tremor was unusually evident. As with our previous meeting, I found the nurse very focused and efficient but rather lacking in empathy. She concentrated almost exclusively on the deficits in my condition and there was no real acknowledgement of my efforts to minimise them. I made it clear that I wanted to have some control over my medication and was insistent that I should be allowed to take the occasional diazepam to enable me to enjoy a social life. She clearly favoured instead alternative methods of relaxation but what I need is very occasional fast-acting medication. I was encouraged to join a trial for a drug that was thought to reduce one's propensity to fall. I agreed to defer any decision until I had read more about it, but the fact that it involves travelling to the Western General Hospital, and that I might well only be given a placebo, makes me reluctant to commit myself too readily.

On the political front, there is mounting evidence of the damage to the economy of recent events. According to the IMF, in 2023 the British economy will be the worst performing of all the advanced economies, with a projected fall of 0.6% in GDP.

It was announced today that the virulent avian flu virus is spreading to animals. There must be a real worry that in the process of crossing species, a new hybrid may emerge capable of infecting humans. The official line is that there is no immediate threat to public health, but we have heard such reassuring noises before!

9th February

Some health issues this week have added new challenges. My bowel movements have become very irregular, and I suspect I will need to increase my daily dose of CosmoCol. To add to my woes, my skin appears to be allergic to the patches that have been so effective in reducing my dribbling. I need to explore whether there is an alternative way of using Hyoscine.

A&E waiting times in Scotland continue to deteriorate. In the final months of 2022 only 62% of patients in A&E were seen and either admitted, transferred or discharged within four hours, as compared with the Scottish Government's target of 95%. It is estimated that in 2022 more than 250 patients needlessly died due to excess waiting times in Scotland's emergency wards.

Meanwhile, we are presented with a political farce in which both Johnson and Truss continue to behave as though their resignations in no way disbar them from interfering in domestic and foreign policy. Truss has continued to argue that her economic policy was correct and shows not a flicker of repentance for the chaos and financial crisis produced by her premiership. Boris is travelling the world as though he is Foreign Secretary. As a result, Rishi Sunak's task of recovering public confidence in the Tory Party is compromised by the sniping of his own backbenchers. North of the Border, Sturgeon has her own cross to bear with Alex Salmond accusing her of putting the cause of Scottish independence back for years by her close involvement with the issue of gender recognition.

The earthquake in Turkey and Syria has left apocalyptic scenes of death and destruction, of homelessness and destitution. Very sadly, the World Health Organisation predicts that more people may die from the aftermath of the earthquake from disease and starvation than from the quake itself.

Three lovely long-tailed tits on the feeders today.

11th February

My computer is clearly on its last legs. For no apparent reason it simply went haywire today and soaked up my time for hours trying to fix it. Fortunately, it has recovered enough for me to save all the folders and files on my desktop and with luck I will not have lost anything. However, I must get a new computer as soon as feasible.

I learnt today that my goddaughter, Susie, had recently got married in a quiet wedding with just two witnesses.

16th February

Yesterday marked a turning point in Scottish politics with the resignation of Nicola Sturgeon. Her leadership had been the subject of increasing criticism in recent weeks from within the SNP as well as from the Scottish media. Although she presented her resignation as a function of fatigue, it was her needless involvement in the gender realignment debate that appears to have been the catalyst for her decision. Her failure to sort out the crisis in the ferry transport sector, and growing evidence of maladministration of public funds by the SNP, added to public disquiet. Above all, recent polls suggested that on the issue of independence the 'yes' vote lagged by 12 points and that Nicola would fail to realise her constitutional ambitions anytime soon. The problem now is that Nicola has never groomed a successor and there is a dearth of real talent in the SNP to take over the leadership. Heaven forfend that Alex Salmond should make yet another come-back from his ALBA Party!

21st February

Not a good week health-wise. Initially, my main issue was pain in my teeth and face that at times was just a dull ache but at other times severe discomfort in my face. I had to resort to pain killers and steam inhalation which has eased the problem, but I suspect this is just another complication of Parkinson's Disease and may well recur. Another problem that has re-emerged is constipation that has recently become a serious issue leaving me feeling nauseous and lacking any appetite. In addition, I have had to cease using the Scoboderm patches as it was clear that they were producing an allergic reaction. Sadly, I have had to defer any visit to Vane Farm until I feel more robust.

News from Suffolk is not good. Apparently my brother is still having fainting episodes and periods of confusion, exacerbated by his hearing impairment. He cannot be left on his own and this must be a real challenge for my sister-in-law. It is so sad that their final years are so blighted.

This Friday marks the anniversary of Putin's invasion of Ukraine. It is anticipated that Putin, Biden and Xi Jinping will all make major speeches that will ramp up their respective commitments to the war. Biden has visited Kiev and reasserted the support of the USA for 'as long as it takes' for Ukraine to recover its territory. However, there is a growing concern within the Republican Party, shared by some Democrats, at the prospect of an endless drain on American military and financial resources. This concern has been fuelled by the view of some military experts that the war may be prolonged for many years, especially now China appears to be contemplating a more active role in supporting Putin's agenda.

Meanwhile, there are ominous signs that the avian flu virus can cross species, with evidence of outbreaks in Spanish mink. Health organisations have stepped up surveillance. Humans can contract avian flu and get sick or even die but the virus would have to change in some way before it could become highly contagious among humans. The fear is that the risk of contagion may rise if a strain of avian virus mixes with another that is more human friendly – a process called genetic re-assortment. Unfortunately, the flu virus is excellent at mutating and recombining. Hopefully, our virologists are on the case!!

26th February

The threat from avian flu has indeed hit the headlines. Although there is still no evidence of human-to-human transference, the possibility that this will occur is sufficiently real that the British Health Security Agency has called for immediate procedures to anticipate any human pandemic.

My health has not been good: further loss of mobility, nausea, loss of appetite and constant problems with my bowel. I have given up the patches as I was clearly allergic to them, and I was concerned at some of their listed side-effects. I am doubling my CosmoCol to regularise my bowel movements. This is all very frustrating as I have had to defer my birdwatching to Vane Farm.

5th March

The political scene is one of implosion, both in the Tories and the SNP. Partygate has reared its ugly head again with the likelihood that the Common's Privileges Committee will find Boris guilty on four counts of misleading the House. If his behaviour is found sufficiently egregious, in theory they could compel a new election in his constituency. Meanwhile, the behaviour and decisions of ministers during the height of the pandemic, of Matt Hancock in particular, has been further called in question by the leak of a mass of WhatsApp messages to the *Daily Telegraph* in Scotland, I suspect in time the behaviour of Nicola and the SNP will be seen to have been equally egregious.

I have struggled with my Parkinson's this past week. In particular, I often feel faint after breakfast.

The real achievement of the week was the success of Mo's play at the Lyceum. She has found it very tiring, but it has done a great deal to boost her self-confidence and to tap into her 'inner thespian'. Our book group met for a discussion of Kate Clanchy's book, *Some kids I taught and what they taught me*. Much to my surprise, most of the group endorsed the view that it contained inappropriate language, albeit her treatment by her publisher and the press had been unacceptable. Our next book, *The Identity Crisis* by Ben Elton, is a wide-ranging satire on political correctness, including issues relating to sex, gender, and race. It is an apt choice given the current melt-down of the SNP over gender recognition, the recent harassment by trans-activists of Hannah Barnes for her exposé of the Tavistock Gender Clinic, and the determination of 'woke', self-appointed cultural gatekeepers to censor the works of Roald Dahl. I was struck by the weariness of the group after three years of the pandemic. Almost all of us had struggled with health problems and remarkably four out of seven of the group had suffered from broken ankles!

Just watched a live streaming of our grandson's ice hockey match; very impressive and delightful to see him in action. Canada really does provide wonderful resources for its kids and the infrastructure that enables them to develop their athletic abilities. Both grandchildren have really exploited these opportunities to the full with their karate and hockey.

12th March

In general, the last week has not been a cheerful experience. Both Mo and I have had colds and, added to my nausea, this has made for poor appetite and fitful sleep. In addition, having stopped my patches, I have had to contend again with constant dribbling; a really unsavoury side-effect of Parkinson's. Meanwhile, the energy price hike has eventually caught up with us with a gas bill over a thousand pounds. Goodness only knows how people on low incomes or dependent on state pensions are going to cope!

Outwith the tedious hustings for a new SNP leader and the febrile debate over the new Immigration Bill, three issues have surfaced of existential significance: The growing trend of intelligence agencies to attribute the source of the pandemic to a Chinese laboratory rather than a 'wet market', the renewed shelling of the energy infrastructure of the nuclear plant in Ukraine, and the insolvency of the Silicon Valley Bank, the biggest bank failure since the 2008 financial crash.

13th March

The ultimate irony! Having survived the pandemic since the first lockdown and diary entry on 19th March 2020, both Mo and I today tested positive for Covid-19. To date, our symptoms have been no worse than a heavy cold and a loss of taste and appetite, together with low energy and a low emotional threshold.

As I feared, the initial assurances from the Government that the UK financial system and tech start-up enterprises were not at serious risk from the collapse of the Silicon Valley Bank was not sufficient to avert a sharp fall on the FTSE. It is to be hoped that the HSBC bail-out will calm the markets.

15th March

The hustings surrounding the selection of a new leader for the SNP have been deeply depressing. The Finance Secretary, deemed economically illiterate by many commentators, appears to be the favoured choice of the general public. However, the SNP membership is currently expected to choose Humza Yousaf, despite the fact that he has a dismal record of non-achievement in a succession of ministerial posts. As one labour MSP unkindly, but accurately observed, Yousaf is 'a charming individual but has all the depth of a summer puddle'.

16th March

Jeremy Hunt's budget yesterday lacked any real attempt to 'level up' British society. While the bulk of the population is in dire straits with the energy, food, and interest rate hikes, the top 1% have been given a huge tax break by the abolition of a cap on pension contributions. While Hunt blithely asserted that the economic prospects were positive, in fact the Office of Budget Responsibility has predicted that over the next two years UK growth performance will be severely constrained and will be accompanied by the biggest fall in real household incomes (some 5.7%) since the 1950s.

The money markets continue to be worryingly volatile following the failure of the Silicon Valley Bank and the dramatic fall in the share price of Credit Suisse. Fears that the economy might be on the edge of another '2008-style crisis' led yesterday to a fall of 293 points in the FTSE; the worst single day since the early days of the pandemic.

Equally worrying is my weight loss. I weighed under eleven stone this morning, the lowest I have been for decades. I clearly need to change my eating habits and closely monitor my weight to make sure there is nothing sinister underlying this.

18th March

Mo has now tested negative for Covid-19 but, as of yesterday, my results still indicated a strong positive viral condition. Both of us are feeling very tired.

The money markets continued to fall on Friday despite reassurances from the US Treasury and EU Bank. Clearly, the initial fears that the collapse of the Silicon Valley Bank might prove contagious was very justified. A lot depends on what happens to Credit Suisse. Irrespective of the outcome, investors have lost massive amounts even if depositors have been protected and the financial viability of the much-hyped tech sector has been called into question.

23rd March

Tested negative today for Covid-19. So far, the symptoms have been no worse than a cold and a few days feeling under par and a loss of energy. My main issue at the moment is my loss of taste, which is having a significant impact on my appetite and weight.

The money markets appear to have settled for the time being but the Bank of England is faced with a serious dilemma. While it wants to raise the bank rate further to counteract inflation, it is precisely the rise in interest rates that have undermined the financial integrity of the tech start-ups. Official figures for the year up to the end of February indicate that, despite the best efforts of the Bank, inflation has continued to rise to 10.4%, with foodstuffs rising by around 18%; inflation rates that have not been experienced since 1977.

Yesterday, Boris performed for several hours before the Commons' Privileges Committee. Opinion is divided as to what the outcome may be, but many political commentators believe that this may be a turning point in Westminster and will scotch any political ambitions, such as a comeback to the premiership, that he may still harbour.

28th March

Mo is due for a colonoscopy today and is naturally very anxious that nothing sinister be discovered. We are both now negative for Covid-19. I am conscious of how far the pandemic has been normalised thanks to the various vaccines. Two years ago, our reaction to a positive test would have been very different, the virus then being feared as a potential life-changer. Today you would struggle to find any coverage of the pandemic in the newspapers, so the degree of risk assessment in our everyday lives has markedly shifted. Covid-19 no longer dominates the political agenda. Gradually, our medical centre is reviving basic treatments such as ear syringing, although there remains a scandalous delay in access to GP appointments. Meanwhile, we are fortunate to be registered with a dental practice given that many have refused to take on additional patients. Even so, much of our treatment now is costed at private rates that far exceed pre-pandemic charges. In many ways the pandemic has widened the inequalities in society with medical, dental, and mental health provisions increasingly a function of wealth rather than need. Anecdotal evidence of Ukrainian refugees returning to their homeland to access treatment only reinforces the belief that our NHS is not fit for purpose.

Putin has further escalated hostilities by threatening to locate tactical nuclear weapons in Belarus. Meanwhile, Trump is inciting riot in the USA as a means of avoiding prosecution and mobilising his right-wing supporters in his re-election bid. Along with the continuing instability in the money markets, the world feels far from secure.

30th March

We have just been referred to a new podcast *Movers and Shakers*, launched by a retired judge and a small group of former BBC journalists and presenters, all of whom have Parkinson's disease. It promises to be an excellent source of information and support.

Developments in Scottish politics are beyond parody! The newly elected SNP leader and First Minister, Humza Yousaf, comes with a dismal track record in a succession of departments – Health, Transport, and Justice. Moreover, in forming his cabinet, he has alienated Kate Forbes, the erstwhile Finance Secretary, who was in my opinion, the only economically half-literate member of Sturgeon's team. Instead, he has appointed Shona Robison, who has never dealt with economic affairs and who was previously sacked as Health Secretary, to be both Finance Secretary and Deputy First Minister. Meanwhile, Angela Constance has been appointed Justice Minister despite her previous removal from both the education and communities and social security portfolios. To compound his incompetence, Yousaf has done away with the post of Transport Secretary (unbelievable given the parlous state of Scottish roads and ferries) and created a publicly funded Minister for Independence, a departure that will inevitably and rightly be challenged in the courts.

A dismal statistic buried in the Sunday papers: Some 30% of children in the UK under the age of 18 are living in 'relative poverty'.

6th April

The SNP is in total disarray after the arrest of its former Chief Executive, Peter Murrell, in relation to the financial affairs of the Party. He has subsequently been released without charge, but it looks as though a whole can of worms is about to be opened. Rumours surrounding the disappearance of £600,000 have long been circulating and the question will inevitably arise as to how far Nicola Sturgeon's resignation as First Minister was triggered by prior knowledge of a likely prosecution.

8th April

The SNP is unravelling at a rate of knots with its auditors now resigning from their role. Rumours of financial misconduct are rife.

I am increasingly concerned about Mo. Ever since the Ballater debacle she has been very tired and stressed. I have spoken to Hilary about the need for Mo to have a break without worrying about me.

We have, however, made real progress in purchasing a new car – a Honda Jazz Cross Star self-charging, automatic hybrid. It will be a steep learning curve for Mo but she found her test drive very enjoyable. I shall miss the VW Golf-plus. It served us well and made the journey to our caravan at Sandgreen a pleasant drive, but it was beginning to show its age and our confidence in its reliability was starting to wane.

13th April

Since my last entry we have made progress towards addressing Mo's needs and have set in place some provisions enabling her to take occasional breaks. Our friends have been very supportive.

On the political front, some Tory MPs have become so disenchanted with the behaviour of their party in Westminster, and its consequent slump in the opinion polls, that they have ceased to issue their local election leaflets in blue! In Scotland, chaos continues to reign within the SNP, and Humza (widely referred to in Holyrood as 'Humza Useless') appears to be faced with an impossible task to reunite the party.

Incredibly, given all the major issues of transport, health, education and the cost of living that require his urgent attention, he has chosen to prioritise a legal challenge to the Government's block on the Gender Recognition Reform Bill. The Bill has already played a major part in dividing the SNP, alienating much of public opinion, and perhaps contributing to Nicola Sturgeon's resignation as First Minister. It is outrageous how Stonewall and trans activists have been allowed to hijack social politics and cultural life in the United Kingdom; even to the extent that in the Lyceum theatre programme for a recent performance of Kidnapped, the cast were listed together with their woke pronouns such as (he/him), (she/her), (she/them), and (they/them). It is absolute nonsense and this form of insidious identity politics needs to be firmly resisted.

For the first time since we moved to Eskbank in 2013 I have heard and sighted a chiffchaff in the garden.

21ˢᵗ April

An eventful week that encompassed a visit to RSPB Loch Leven and a National Theatre filmed performance. Paul and I enjoyed a very productive day at Vane Farm, viewing over twenty bird species including a marsh harrier. The weather was perfect for bird watching and, out of the wind, certainly the warmest day of the year so far. The play 'Good' was superb, with an outstanding performance by David Tennant, newly returned to the London stage.

Breaking news; Dominic Raab, the Deputy Prime Minister, has resigned after an investigation upheld accusations of his previous bullying behaviour in a number of departments. Not the whitewash I had predicted !

Meanwhile, the British economy appears to be locked into slow growth and high inflation; the latter remaining at above 10% with food costs rising at around 19%. The Bank of England is almost certainly going to raise the Bank Rate further to control inflation, but this in turn will constrain investment.

For the moment the pandemic has disappeared from the headlines. There are occasional references to the incidence of infection but for the most part it is now treated as a normal fact of life. Indeed, so much so that my recent booster vaccination did not even merit a diary entry. However, an Omicron sub-variant – XBB.1.16 or Arcturus – has emerged in India and has now spread to 28 countries including the UK. It appears to be highly transmissible but, to date, no more serious in its effects than previous variants. One to watch methinks!

23rd April

The Sunday papers are replete with dire predictions of the fall of the SNP and the lost cause of Scottish independence. Editorials have focused on the rapid erosion of Nicola's reputation and the growing disenchantment within the SNP at the legacy she has left. Surreal images of police digging up her garden, evoking memories of Fred and Rose West, have only served to add to the sense of unreality surrounding recent developments. As the erstwhile, self-styled 'continuity candidate' for the post of First Minister Humza looks increasingly beleaguered.

25th April

Yesterday, I had my second ever tooth extraction. My first one was many years ago due to the criminal malpractice of the Mitchell brothers; dentists who operated in Edinburgh and the borders who conned patients into having expensive and needless treatments and did untold damage to patients' dental health. They were subsequently exposed in a 'Checkpoint' programme on Channel 4. Curiously, while a recent filling cost several hundred pounds, the extraction only cost some £18. This is because my filling did not fall under the remit of the NHS and was subject to a private tariff. I feel very fortunate to have been able to access any NHS treatment, as across the UK nine out of ten dental practices are no longer undertaking NHS work and only undertaking private work.

The optics surrounding the SNP grow increasingly toxic. Humza is reputedly now being called 'LINO'.(Leader In Name Only)! Meanwhile, the investigation into its finances has revealed that several SNP officials possessed 'burner' phones, evoking memories of *The Wire*.

30th April

A rare garden sighting today of a pair of goldfinches. For some reason they have rarely visited my feeders. In addition, a series of raucous cries turned out to be gulls dive-bombing a magnificent Grey Heron that sat imposingly on our garage roof, no doubt scanning our small pond for signs of life.

I managed to walk ten circuits of the garden to get some fresh air and to try and strengthen my legs. The *Movers and Shakers* podcast has confirmed the importance for Parkinson's sufferers of exercise for stamina and balance and I must pursue this. My feeling is that having a personal trainer and one-to-one sessions would be the most effective option.

7th May

A watershed moment this week as the World Health Organisation announced that Covid-19 no longer constituted a 'global health emergency'. Nevertheless, the full extent of long Covid has yet to be recognised and properly addressed. Certainly, Covid-related ill-health is impacting on absenteeism in the workforce.

We watched the coronation yesterday of Charles 3rd. It was a magnificent spectacle and more emotional than I had anticipated. I fully appreciate how many people view the monarchy as an expensive and archaic indulgence, but it is difficult to think of anyone who one would trust as a President.

The Conservatives have been soundly and rightly trounced in the English local elections. However, election pundits caution that Labour's performance would not necessarily translate at a General Election into a comfortable working majority. Keir Starmer still struggles to come across as a dynamic and inspiring leader. His forensic style lacks charisma. He also seems prone to silly and avoidable gaffs. Who on earth, given the history of antisemitism in the party, persuaded him to label Labour activists as his 'Starmtroopers'!

The international news has mainly centred on Sudan where warring factions have created a 'humanitarian catastrophe'. Ukraine has also resurfaced in the media with the impending spring offensive and continued concerns over the safety of the nuclear plant at Zaporizhzhia.

My Parkinson's has really deteriorated over the last week, and I am struggling to move my feet. I suspect that I need to do more exercises. It could also be due to my preoccupation with transitioning to a new computer as IT issues have a way of weighing on my mind and inhibiting the synapses I need for moving about.

12th May

My Parkinson's continues to give me grief. Although I have had success in dealing with low blood pressure and constipation, my balance has seriously deteriorated, as has my proclivity for 'sticking' and festination. However, we have taken some steps to acquire a personal trainer to try and improve my coordination. This weekend Mo is taking a much-needed break in York, presuming that the current railway strikes do not abort arrangements. Various people are going to check up on me and/or take me out.

Some worrying items in the news. Another bank has become insolvent in the United States reviving fears of 'contagion' in the money markets. Meanwhile, Britain has begun to supply Ukraine with ballistic missiles, risking a dangerous escalation in the level of hostilities. Finally, despite Trump being found guilty of sexual assault and harassment, political commentators consider that his previous supporters will dismiss the allegations as spurious and vote for his reinstatement as President.

We await the final of the European Song Contest with little expectation that the UK will win. It is a mystery how boringly banal our contribution is, given the singing and song-writing talent that we have in this country.

We have certainly been unlucky with our next-door neighbours who assail us with constant drilling, the smell of dope, and intermittent incidents involving aggressive swearing in the street and heavy police presence. Unfortunately, there is little we can do to rectify the situation. They are clearly running a business from home contrary to their title deeds, but we are advised that it is unlikely that we could obtain any sort of court order. Moreover, they have no sense of social civilities, and any complaint is likely to induce even worse egregious behaviour. It is perhaps apposite that the arrival of such a 'maverick' family was facilitated by *Purple Bricks*, a down-market online estate agency that was valued at £1.5 billion in 2017 but is today insolvent and worthless!

14th May

Yesterday, while Mo is away in York for a break, I was taken to Innerleithen for an afternoon on my scooter in the sun. The temperature was just right and the scenery superb and hugely relaxing. I spotted sand martins skittering over the riverbanks collecting mud to line their nests. Also, a brief and rare sighting of a pied flycatcher and a curious plethora of orange tip butterflies! My mobility using the walker was dire and my bladder played its usual tricks but otherwise a wonderful day, not least because Hilary and Martin were so patient and attentive. I was very struck by a quote I read today from Edmund Burke, the 18th century statesman and philosopher, that seemed to have especial relevance to British politics today:

'Rage and frenzy will pull down more in half-an-hour, than prudence, deliberation and foresight can build up in a hundred years. Something for our political leaders to take on board!'

27th May

We are faced with a somewhat stressful week leading up to our week's break in Kirkcudbright. Due to a delivery cock-up my new computer has yet to be delivered and set up. Meanwhile, with the MOT due on our Golf Plus on 4th June we are still awaiting delivery of our new car. Thankfully, the weather is very warm and it has been delightful to sit in the garden and listen to the birdsong while the bluetits feed on the aphids that are taking over our roses. Using the scooter on the lawn as a seat works very well and provides me with more security than struggling with a wobbly chair.

I have begun to undertake the exercises suggested by my 'personal trainer'. Combined with my existing routine, this gives me a solid work-out. However, I need to be aware that the leg exercises leave me unstable later in the day.

12th June

An eventful few days since my last entry. Our break in Kirkcudbright was blessed with very fine weather, albeit there was often more hazy sunshine in the mornings than the BBC forecast predicted. The apartment was in a good location but poorly furnished and equipped. As always, the scenery was beautiful, with the whin and hawthorn in full colour. Our birdwatching plans were frustrated by the temporary closure for renovation of several hides. The exception was the hide at Kirroughtree that yielded a great sighting of the Great Spotted Woodpecker, along with a nuthatch and a lively red squirrel.

Meanwhile, the legacy of the pandemic continues to shape British politics. Faced with a damning report on his behaviour from the Commons Privilege Committee, Johnson has resigned amidst turmoil within the Tory Party, triggering a bye-election that is likely to add further to what one reviewer has dubbed 'the post-Brexit Tory psychodrama'. North of the Border, the SNP are in similar disarray, Nicola Sturgeon having been arrested for questioning in connection with the finances of the Party.

The origins of the pandemic have also become again a focus for public debate. It appears that in 2019, at the Institute of Virology in Wuhan, scientists and the Chinese military were combining a deadly cocktail of Coronaviruses to create a new mutant strain. Evidence suggests that there was some form of leakage leading to the hospitalisation of laboratory workers as early as November 2019, that was not publicised.

21st June

A slight hiatus in my diary entry to accommodate the acquisition of a new hybrid car and a new MacBook Pro, both of which will entail a fairly steep learning curve. Much to my delight most of the important files transferred from my old computer, albeit only after I employed a specialist to set up my machine. Even better, my loyal laser printer, that has seen me through many a book and article, can still be used.

The fallout from the report of the Privileges Committee continues to occupy Westminster. A Common's vote overwhelmingly endorsed its condemnation of Boris Johnson after an outstanding debate that rightly addressed the impact of his egregious behaviour on the reputation of Parliament. Sadly, the Prime Minister did not feel fit to attend.

The pandemic continues to lurk in the background. Clearly, many people with long Covid are still very unwell and the impact of the lockdowns on mental health, especially in the young, is only now being properly acknowledged. Conspiracy theories relating to the origins and management of the pandemic have resurfaced with a vengeance in recent weeks and the proceedings of the Committee on the handling of the virus promise to keep the pandemic prominent in public discourse.

My Parkinson's is making life a real struggle. Some days I can barely move my legs and every task takes forever. In addition, my constant dribbling is hugely depressing, and I intend to consult the Parkinson's nurses as to an alternative medication.

22nd June

The news was dominated today by yet another rise in the Bank Rate, adding to the cost-of-living crisis for thousands of families. We spent the day in Innerleithen with great weather. The amount of foliage made bird watching difficult but enroute I spotted a red kite and by the riverbanks heard the distinctive reeling sound of a grasshopper warbler. Sadly, the sand martins appeared to have departed.

23rd June

Not a good day. My movements and dribbling were dire and I could barely play my guitar. My brain appeared to have little connection to my limbs.

Today was the 7th anniversary of Brexit, the most egregious act of national self-harm that is still hampering British trade and industry and dividing society. Yet another legacy of a corrupt and self-seeking Government that deluded the electorate.

26th June

Exciting times. The news is dominated by the mutiny (? failed coup) in Russia of the mercenary Wagner Group and its possible repercussions for the future of Putin. At home, Elton John's final UK performance last night at Glastonbury was sensational.

29th June

The evidence before the Covid Inquiry is revealing the absence of any effective preparation for a pandemic. Hancock has argued that, in the early months of 2020, British policy makers panicked and initially focused on the immediate effects of a pandemic such as the likely shortage of body bags rather than the best strategy for containing the virus.

The bulk of the Wagner Group are now exiled in Belarus, forming an unpredictable and destabilising force in the region. It remains to be seen how far Putin's position has been permanently compromised. The podcast *Battleground Ukraine* is proving invaluable in interpreting events.

5th July

Last week was a period of relative calm after the rather hectic acquisition of a new car and new computer. Both are proving a blessing. I have managed to install Skype but still struggling with the University guidelines for Zoom. I have felt under par the last few days and, despite drinking plenty of water, had a light-headed incident this morning. It will be good to catch up with my consultant next week; our first face-to-face meeting in 3 years!

I am finding that a combination of podcasts plus *The Week* magazine provides me with an excellent overview of British and world news including developments in Ukraine. Both in Westminster and Holyrood, the personal misdemeanours of our legislators continue to distract the policy community from addressing key social and economic issues and to starve the body politic of oxygen. Existential threats such as climate change and the likelihood of another pandemic are met with vague and unconvincing sound bites. Issues that cry out for a cross-party consensual approach are instead 'weaponised' to score cheap political points.

I have been updating my 'Final Wishes' briefing note for Mo, a somewhat depressing task but needs must. It is surprisingly difficult to select music that is neither too doom-laden nor inappropriately rousing. I have to keep reminding myself that I am NOT going to be there, and it is the likely impact of the music on the mourners that matters!

7th July

Some interesting news from Ukraine. It appears that the Ukrainian forces may be about to retake Bakhmut after encircling Russian troops. If this is so, it will be a major advance in the counter-offensive. Less encouraging is the Russian accusation that the Ukrainians are planning to blow up the nuclear power plant at Zaporizhzhia. It seems an improbable claim but the very fact that it is part of the ongoing narrative is deeply disturbing, as is the possibility that some 700,000 children have been separated from their families and deported from the occupied Ukrainian territories to Russia.

10th July

Rishi Sunak's five pledges appear increasingly untenable. There is no let-up to the arrival of immigrants in small boats. The economy is flatlining, core inflation remains high and national debt has hit 100% of GDP. Unsurprisingly, polls indicate that Labour is as much as 25 points ahead of the Conservative Party. However, the shift in UK politics in favour of Labour runs counter to a worrying rise of far-right nationalist parties across Europe. In Germany, the 'Alternative for Germany' anti-immigrant party has gained ground in municipal elections, led by Alice Weidel who espouses neo-Nazi views. In Italy, the nationalist Giorgia Meloni has been installed as Prime Minister. Finland has the most right-wing government in its history and hard-right parties are also flourishing in Greece and Sweden.

15th July

My annual consultation with Dr Davenport went well. He was very focused and supportive and made a point of affirming the positive role my mental attitude had played in coping with Parkinson's. He is going to prescribe new medications for my festination and dribbling to see whether they might make a difference, although he observed that, to date, there was nothing that could specifically target my freezing and poor balance.

Our dystopian neighbours surpassed themselves last night, with loud and aggressive shouting followed by items being thrown at our conservatory and into our garden. As a result, we felt compelled to call the police. Fortunately, they have put their house on the market with a view to moving to a more rural location where the son's behaviour will be less evident. We shall be mightily relieved when they go.

21st July

There were several positives this week. Our neighbours are beginning to receive viewers and hopefully will secure a speedy sale. Certainly, everything has gone very quiet since the last incident. I do hope any newcomers are not dog lovers as I would dearly like to have another cat. It is over two years since we lost our poor Bella.

My consultant's report covered all the issues raised during my recent appointment and he has set out a range of options to try and address my mobility and dribbling issues. I was somewhat heartened by his aside that I 'remained more active than many men of my age even without a neurodegenerative disease'! I took the initiative and booked *The Black Ivy* for my birthday lunch. The staff were really supportive, and the hotel has excellent disabled access. I look forward to using it as a regular meeting place in the future.

The outcome of the three by-elections looks promising. If one discards the narrow Tory win in Uxbridge and South Ruislip that was primarily a protest vote against the proposed extension of the London Ultra Low Emissions Zone, the other results indicate a swing of over 20% away from the Government. However, most commentators were predicting a clean sweep and the outcome suggests that the cost of green initiatives can have real traction on local politics.

News from Ukraine suggests that it continues to be a war of attrition. The most notable development this week has been the Ukrainian attack on the Kerch Bridge that joins Russia to the occupied Crimea: very much a symbol of Russian expansionism.

1st August

The weather is dismal and dreich and the summer appears to have disappeared, ironic given that June was declared the warmest month across the world since records began. Indeed, climatologists consider that the temperatures now being recorded were last experienced over 150,000 years ago!

I am starting a new exercise routine drawn up by my 'personal trainer' and designed to increase my strength, coordination, alignment and balance. I suspect it will take me some time to transition to a new schedule, but I think it will help me remain active and positive. I have also added Amitriptyline to my medications in the hope that it might reduce my dribbling. Meanwhile, additional medication for my festination and freezing has still to be resolved between my GP and consultant.

Although the pandemic is for now marginalised in the media, the impact of long Covid on the work force and the NHS is increasingly evident. A vast number of people are claiming unemployment benefit due to the physical and mental after-effects of the virus and lockdowns. Conspiracy theories still surround the causes of Covid-19.

Trump has now been indicted for his attempts to invalidate Biden's election to President, for his interference in the election process and for his incitement of his supporters to riot at the Capitol in January 2021. He has openly declared that he can become President even if he is found guilty in current criminal proceedings against him. The prospect of the USA self-destructing with civil rioting in 2024 is very real, as is the likelihood that, in the event of a Trump victory, American support for Ukraine would be reappraised.

8ᵗʰ August

My dribbling continues unabated, and I may have to switch from Amitriptyline to Atropine eye drops in line with my consultant's advice A fall last night has unnerved me. Fortunately, I do not appear to have broken anything but inevitably it plays with my mind and undermines my confidence. Unfortunately, it is virtually impossible to gain access to my GP in the foreseeable future, even just a telephone call, to discuss my medication.

The Tory immigration 'gong show' is back in town! The latest initiative, (risibly promoted by Sunak as part of his 'Small Boats Week'), is to decamp asylum seekers from hotels to coastal barges while their cases are processed as a deterrent to those seeking to cross the channel illegally. The Home Office is struggling to fill just one barge off the Dorset coast, the Bibby Stockholm, with 500 immigrants, while across the country there are 50,000 immigrants still housed in hotel accommodation. In addition, under the powers conveyed by the Illegal Immigration Bill, it is intended that, in future, subject to a favourable ruling from the Supreme Court, such immigrants will be extradited to Rwanda (or perhaps even the Ascension Islands!) to have their cases assessed. Like so much of the Home Office's proposals, it is all beyond parody, especially when it is estimated that there is a backlog of some 170,000 asylum applications still awaiting to be processed.

More hopeful is the news that a new Vaccine Development and Evaluation Centre is to open on the Porton Down Campus to prepare for future pandemics and to target existing diseases with a high mortality rate, such as the tic-borne virus Crimean-Congo haemorrhagic fever, that are spreading into Europe, as a consequence of global warming.

11th August

Postscript: Just to add to Sunak's woes, the Bibby Stockholm has had to be evacuated due to the discovery of Legionella bacteria in its water supply.

18th August

Still struggling with my mobility and constant dribbling. I have tried to obtain fresh medication but there are communication problems between my GP and consultant that have delayed matters. Another 'light-headed' episode this morning despite drinking lots of water. Perhaps I need to reduce my food intake at breakfast.

The debate over the initial source of the pandemic has resurfaced in recent weeks. It appears that within US intelligence and Republican circles there is a growing belief that the origins of the pandemic lay in a leak from the Wuhan Institute of Virology where 'gain of function' experiments were being carried out on infected bats, partly funded by the US government. The WHO inspection of the Wuhan Institute is regarded as having been wholly inadequate. Meanwhile, there are reports of a new Omicron variant that is reported to be highly infectious.

The war in Ukraine remains in deadlock with the Russian defences slowing down the Ukrainian counter-offensive. Meanwhile, the Black Sea has now become a major area of conflict with NATO and the US threatening direct military intervention if Russia seeks to control the waterways.

28th August

Back at home after a very pleasant week in Pittenweem in an apartment overlooking the sea, culminating in a thoroughly indulgent meal in the Dory Bistro, including lobster. The weather was warm and sunny throughout our stay. We had two very successful excursions, a wonderful visit to Cambo gardens with its spectacular display of garden and wild flowers and a brief, but very successful couple of hours in the Eden Nature Reserve just outside St Andrews. We were rewarded with a view of an osprey, a little egret, a ruff, and several kingfishers.

An eventful week on the international front with the death of the Wagner leader, Prigozhin, in an air crash; almost certainly a planned assassination. On the ground, Ukrainian forces are gaining some ground and beginning to breach the Russian defences. Elsewhere, two developments do not augur well for the future; the increasing likelihood that Trump with end up in the White House rather than the jailhouse, and the ominous crash in property values in China that may drag the world economy into another financial crisis.

On the home front, there is news of a new Omicron variant BVA2.86, named Pirola. It is apparently no more serious in its medical effects but is worryingly capable of a much higher number of mutations.

Mo is increasingly reluctant to get another cat. I can appreciate her concerns, but I find the thought that we will never have another furry friend very depressing!

5th September

So far, very little information on the Pirola virus but the World Health Organisation has deemed it a development 'of interest' and in recent weeks the number of Covid-related hospitalisations and deaths in the UK has witnessed an upswing, albeit they remain a fraction of previous levels.

The Government remains in disarray. The number of illegal immigrants crossing the channel has been boosted by the good weather. The level of inflation, bank rate, and national debt all remain ominously high, and a major scandal has broken over the structural safety of the nation's schools. Indeed, some commentators are predicting that the sudden closure of schools on the eve of term may well be Sunak's 'Poll Tax' moment. Meanwhile, Birmingham, the second largest city in Europe, has declared itself bankrupt and able to fund only the most basic, statutory services!

I have now added two additional medications to my cocktail of drugs, in an effort to improve my 'connectivity' and reduce my dribbling. In addition, I am endeavouring to exercise in accordance with the advice of my personal trainer.

7th September

We took advantage of the current heatwave to visit Vane Farm for some birdwatching. The weather was perfect but sadly there were very few birds. None of the usual waders were on show. However, there was some consolation in the presence of three ospreys on the distant fence posts. It was also a useful opportunity to use a more truncated scope rest to lighten our load. Clearly, August and September are not ideal for birdwatching at Loch Leven.

11th September

The medical authorities are becoming increasingly concerned about the new variant BVA2.86 (Pirola) which appears to be circulating in the community. Understandably, Edinburgh was the UK's Covid hotspot during the festival. However, it is hard to track its progress as there is so little community testing since free lateral flow tests are no longer available.

I am relieved that both Mo and I have been allocated early slots for flu and Coronavirus vaccinations. The new medication, Atropine Sulphate, appears to be reducing my dribbling. I have also begun to take Rasagiline for my festination and freezing but it will be several weeks before I can assess its value. I now have a broad range of exercises set out by my personal trainer and have begun to take her advice on how to operate my new walker without stress.

18th September

The weather has now become distinctly autumnal and much cooler. The power cleaning of the drive has refreshed the garden and some of the roses are still displaying. However, the crop of apples is a big disappointment: very mushy and not readily cored. Life is rather flat except for the outrageous behaviour of my grandson and his fiancée and the worrying prospect that Mo may need invasive treatment for hyperparathyroidism. No doubt there will be many months of delay before Mo sees a consultant, and further delays thereafter before an operation. There is a possibility that any treatment may have to be private given the protracted delays in NHS elective surgery.

24th September

For some time, news of the war in Ukraine has been somewhat marginalised by natural disasters in Libya and Morocco. However, Ukrainian forces have made important gains on the battlefield, particularly south of Bakhmut and in western Zaporizhia, and successfully degraded Russia's defensive capabilities in the Crimea. They have also targeted Russia's Black Sea fleet using Storm Shadow missiles supplied by the UK and France.

In Britain, the news is dominated by Sunak's sudden dilution of the UK's Net Zero targets and threatened abandonment of various sections of HS2. In addition, he is reviewing the possibility of a reduction and eventual cancellation of Inheritance Tax, despite the fact that it would only benefit the top 4% of wealth holders in the country. He is clearly trying to salvage Tory fortunes in advance of the coming General Election, but today's papers indicate that his proposals will meet strong opposition, especially from industrialists and northern civic leaders who have already invested heavily in infrastructure and renewable technologies.

28th September

Hopefully, Mo's new medication will ease some of the symptoms relating to her hyperparathyroidism while she awaits an appointment with a consultant. My own health is fragile. While my new medication seems to have greatly reduced my dribbling, and my tremor is tolerable, my loss of balance, festination and freezing makes every journey indoors a time-consuming struggle. In addition, I need to be very careful not to lower my blood pressure in the morning as I am prone to feeling faint and momentarily losing consciousness, much to Mo's distress. However, my new walker has enabled me to stroll in the garden non-stop for 1–20 minutes which will hopefully strengthen my legs and enable me to access venues without needing my scooter.

The Tory Government continues unerringly to shoot itself in the foot. Sunak has now not only reneged on his commitment to extend HS2 to Manchester but also given approval for the opening of a new North Sea gas and oil field. Meanwhile, Suella (more aptly Cruella!) Braverman has made an outrageous speech condemning multiculturalism and the international asylum system, and questioning whether being gay and subject to discrimination was sufficient justification for granting asylum.

I note that there is further crisis in the Chinese property market with Evergrande ceasing to trade, and I suspect that it will only be a matter of time before it impacts on the international money markets.

4th October

The news is dominated by the Tory annual conference and the dissension over Rishi Sunak's anticipated pruning back of HS2 and his reluctance to introduce any tax cuts. What is most worrying and inexplicable is the continuing influence of Liz Truss who has become the darling of the far right of the Conservative Party and successfully highjacked proceedings at the conference. Given her catastrophic tenure of the premiership one can only despair at the renewed support for her narcissistic, delusional ideas and ambitions. The re-emergence of Farage at the epicentre of conference proceedings is equally troubling, and there are those in the commentariat who are speculating that he might yet become a future Prime Minister.

The proceedings of the Covid Inquiry on the handling of the pandemic are producing some fascinating evidence. Sir Patrick Valence, formerly the Government Chief Scientific Officer and Sir Chris Whitty, formerly England's CMO, have testified to the chaos and panic in Downing Street as the virus took hold in the early months of 2020 and the failure of Johnson properly to engage with their advice and consult on policy issues relating to the introduction and relaxation of lockdown restrictions. In his diary, Valence described one morning meeting with Johnson as 'complete bollocks' and 'like bipolar decision making'. Later in the year he recorded that it was 'almost impossible' to get agreement on anything due to the civil war within Downing Street and the 'massive internal operational mess' within the Department of Health and Public Health England. In evidence to the Covid Inquiry, Valence emphasised that the scientists had only given advice and not made policy, and he considered that the mantra of 'following the science' had enabled ministers to use him and the CMO as 'human shields' at the press conferences.

Channel 4's dramatization of 'Partygate', based on the Sue Gray report, was a damning indictment of the behaviour of Downing Street staff over the Christmas period of 2020 when the country was in strict lockdown. Some fifteen parties were shown to have taken place in clear contravention of Covid regulations.

8th October

Since my last entry I have had another fall. Fortunately, it was in the conservatory and no real injury was sustained, but it does reflect my deteriorating balance. Reading through my previous diaries I was interested to see that it was a year ago to the day that I suggested to Mo that I would probably need a wheelchair indoors before long. In a way it is a very positive sign that, although we subsequently purchased a chair, it has not yet been needed.

Dreadful news today from the Middle East as a new war has broken out between Israel and the Hamas Palestinian militants. Both sides have suffered many deaths and injuries, and Hamas, an offshoot of the Islamic Brotherhood, has captured scores of Israeli civilians to hold as hostage. As I write, the Israeli forces are unleashing their counterattack on Gaza. The whole incident is being regarded as 'Israel's 9/11'.

The news on the war in Ukraine is also depressing. The counterattack against the Russian forces has recently only made minor gains of territory and it is likely that hostilities will drag on into 2024 at the very least. In addition, there are signs that military support for Ukraine is by no means secure. NATO has warned that its members are fast exhausting their stock of armaments and munitions. Several countries, such as Poland, Slovakia, and Hungary have witnessed a shift in public and political opinion in favour of Russia. More significantly, in the USA, the Republican Party has successfully stalled any new tranche of military aid to Ukraine by their opposition to Biden's budget proposals and their suspension of the Speaker of the House of Representatives.

13th October

Not a good week health wise. Another fall, the second in a week, this time in my study, involving a head injury. Fortunately, despite a sizeable gash in my skull, I did not lose consciousness and had no symptoms of concussion. But it has left me feeling very vulnerable. I seem to have lost my appetite and for the first time since I was diagnosed with Parkinson's I struggle to keep to my routines.

The current Covid Inquiry has revealed that, in the early months of 2020, Downing Street failed to share vital information about the pandemic and failed to involve the devolved administrations in the timing of the first lockdown, whose delay seriously inflated the levels of infection, hospitalisation, and deaths in the community.

As I write, Israel is about to besiege Gaza in response to the massacre and hostage taking carried out by Hamas. One commentator observed that recent events had led to the killing of more Jews than at any time since the Holocaust! The suffering of citizens in Israel and Gaza is hard to imagine and to view on screen.

16ᵗʰ October

The news from the Middle East is horrendous and Gaza is fast becoming a catastrophe, with the prospect of all-out war when Israeli forces finally invade Gaza, in an effort to destroy Hamas once and for all. There is a serious possibility that Hezbollah in Lebanon will also become involved, with support from Iran, precipitating a wider regional conflict.

At home, the proceedings of the Covid-19 Inquiry have revealed the utter chaos in the Cabinet Office in 2020 with Carrie Johnson intervening in policymaking and briefing against the head of the civil service, Simon Case. In his view, expressed in WhatsApp messages to Dominic Cummings, the Government was looking like a 'terrible, tragic joke' and lacked the credibility to impose a lockdown after previously deciding against such a move. As a result, when full lockdown *was* finally imposed, the pandemic had already driven the NHS and the care sector into crisis.

20ᵗʰ October

Further revelations from the Covid-19 Inquiry of the chaotic process of decision making in September 2020. Johnson's scientific advisers were opposed to Rishi Sunak's 'eat out to help out' scheme as likely to increase the spread of the virus. Indeed, the Deputy Chief Scientific Adviser referred to Sunak as 'Doctor Death' in her exchanges with colleagues.

Storm Babet is taking its toll on the North-East. So far, we have escaped the worst of it, but strong winds are scheduled for the rest of the day.

Israeli forces have still not invaded Gaza which is fast becoming a humanitarian disaster, starved of fuel, food, and water. Events in the Middle East have come to dominate the news and podcasts. Meanwhile, the US House of Representatives has still not elected a Speaker, which effectively paralyses the efforts of Biden to send support to both Gaza and Ukraine.

At home, the Labour Party has just won another two by-elections with swings of over twenty percent. This augurs well for the next general election but, on a cautionary note, the by-elections had a very low turnout and there is some evidence that the result reflected the reluctance of Conservative voters to turn out rather than a positive commitment to Labour. However, John Curtice considers that it is a 'seismic event' and could indicate a dramatic fall in Tory fortunes.

24th October

The invasion of Israeli forces into Gaza is still on hold and the world's press remains focused on the atrocities carried out by Hamas, on the plight of the hostages, and on the apocalyptic conditions suffered by the residents of Gaza. Many commentators have warned that this massacre and imminent invasion could easily provide the trigger for a wider war in the Middle East if Hezbollah in Lebanon becomes more involved with the backing of Iran and Syria, drawing a predictable response from American warships anchored off the coast.

At home, many parts of Scotland are still recovering from the flood damage caused by Storm Babet, with more rain forecast. The SNP remain in disarray, displaying their customary economic illiteracy. Their latest proposal to continue to freeze the council tax beggars belief, given that it will further impoverish local authorities and merely add to the cuts already suffered by social services over the last decade.

Health-wise, I continue to suffer from poor balance and freezing. However, I have not had any significant side effects from my vaccinations and my head injury appears to be healing well, albeit I will be left with some scarring. A change in medication has certainly alleviated my problem of dribbling. It remains for me to up my dosage of Co-careldopa to see if I can reduce my episodes of freezing.

Meanwhile, in Ukraine, although the Ukrainian forces have managed to establish a small bridgehead across the Dnieper and to deplete Russian military assets in Eastern Ukraine with recently acquired long-range ballistic missiles (ATACMS), the fighting elsewhere appears to be deadlocked and set to continue through a second winter. Perhaps, most worrying, is the appointment of a new Republican Speaker to the House of Representatives who shares Trump's opposition to continued support for Ukraine.

31st October

We have been avidly following the proceedings of the UK Covid Inquiry into the handling of the pandemic. Clearly, in the first weeks of 2020 there was a failure of Boris Johnson and the Cabinet Office, first to appreciate the significance of the outbreak in Wuhan, and thereafter to formulate a clear and coherent policy for managing the pandemic in the UK. WhatsApp messages reveal that the Cabinet Office was in chaos, with Johnson swithering (or in the parlance of his critics 'trolleying') between alternative strategies, presiding over a 'toxic macho culture', and not in command of the situation. As a result, there was a fatal delay in the imposition of the first lockdown, by which time the levels of infection, hospitalisation, and death within the community were rising exponentially. Later in the year Boris was again resistant to a second lockdown, promoting instead a crude 'herd immunity' notion of letting the virus have free rein amongst the elderly, in order to save the younger workforce and the economy.

9th November

The Covid-19 Inquiry continues to provide compelling evidence of the 'feral' culture over which Boris presided in Downing Street in 2020–2021. Mark Sedwill, former head of the civil service, described Johnson's team as 'brutal and useless'. Watching the proceedings is addictive but a sad commentary on the quality of governance in recent years. Some commentators have questioned whether the adversarial nature of the Inquiry is suited to identifying the lessons to be learned for the future rather than simply distributing blame for the past. It shows no signs of probing the fundamental question of whether the pandemic restrictions were worth the sacrifices they entailed.

The invasion of Gaza is ongoing with the Israeli forces effectively razing the settlement to the ground without any apparent forethought as to where the Palestinian population is going to settle after the war. It is difficult to see any resolution of the situation that will ensure any lasting peace for the region.

My balance and mobility remain a constant issue. However, I have now started on some medication that has greatly reduced my dribbling. In addition, I have increased my Co-careldopa in the hope of reducing my freezing and festination. I have also begun to take the Co-careldopa some 45–60 minutes before eating to optimize its effect, in line with advice on the *Movers and Shakers* podcast. In fact, it is Mo's health that is my greatest concern with the prospect of an operation for hyperparathyroidism and ongoing pains in all her joints that are leaving her tired and stressed.

18th November

An eventful week in both domestic and international affairs. In Ukraine, the Ukrainian forces have established more bridgeheads across the Dnieper and continued to target Russian supply lines. It is estimated that to date up to 300,000 Russian troops have been killed or injured in the war. However, there are signs that NATO is running out of armaments and that events in Gaza are proving a distraction. In the US the Republican Party is increasingly resistant to any open-ended commitment to supplying arms to Ukraine: a view that is strongly endorsed by Trump in his preliminary campaign to win the next presidential election.

Meanwhile, the Israeli invasion of Gaza continues to create a humanitarian disaster with thousands of Palestinians killed or maimed and over a million displaced without housing, food, water, and medical care. At home, the apocalyptic conditions in Gaza have created divisions within the Labour Party. While Keir Starmer has called for a 'humanitarian pause' to the war, many of his shadow cabinet have argued for a 'ceasefire', and either resigned or been sacked from their posts.

The Tories have also had an eventful and divisive week. Despite a Supreme Court ruling against the Rwanda scheme for processing immigrants, Sunak, having sacked Suella Braverman, is determined to proceed with it by means of legislation and a formal treaty with Rwanda, even if this is found contrary to international law. Indeed, there are many on the Tory right wing who are calling for Britain to withdraw from the European Convention on Human Rights and the United Nation's Convention on Refugees to forestall any further legal obstruction to the scheme. Given that, at most, the scheme would process a few hundred immigrants, and that currently the backlog of cases numbers around 175,000, the whole issue is further testimony to the moral and intellectual bankruptcy of the present Government.

The sudden appointment of David Cameron as Foreign Secretary only highlights the incoherence of Sunak's government. Cameron was the Prime Minister who drove the damaging austerity agenda, who made the unrealistic promise to cut annual net migration numbers to below 100,000, who naively invited China to invest in UK nuclear power stations and who called for and lost the Brexit referendum. After leaving office he was involved in highly dubious lobbying for the now bankrupt Greenhill Capital.

23rd November

A busy but successful week taking in a visit to Vane Farm and GD's inaugural lecture. The weather was ideal for birdwatching: cold but still and excellent light. Apart from the usual suspects (teal, golden eye, pochard, widgeon, and gadwall), we saw a stunning whooper swan, three little egrets, and a marsh harrier. The scooter performed well, and PS is always excellent company and hugely supportive.

Gayle's inaugural lecture was a great success. Her autobiographical approach was pitched with humour and clearly captivated the audience, and she was hugely generous in her remarks about my role in her career. We were so proud of her.

The evidence this week presented to the Covid-19 Inquiry by Patrick Vallance and Chris Witty, the Chief Scientific and Medical Officers who dominated the Government's regular press conferences in 2020, has revealed some fascinating insights into 'the bipolar decision making' in the early months of 2020. Clearly, they had been increasingly uneasy about the use of the mantra of 'following the science' as it blurred the distinction between their role as technical advisors and the politicians' responsibility for policy making. Their evidence suggests that at the start of the pandemic Vallance and Witty were by no means in lockstep over their advice on the timing of the first lockdown, with Witty favouring a more cautious approach. In hindsight, both admitted that the delay in introducing lockdown had enabled the pandemic to get out of control and caused additional deaths. Other evidence to the Inquiry has highlighted Boris Johnson's inability to understand the statistical information being presented to the Cabinet. In addition, it transpires that Sunak did not forewarn Witty and Vallance of the introduction of his 'Eat Out to Help Out' scheme later in the year: a scheme that was directly contrary to the ongoing campaign to encourage distancing and masking, and that contributed to the further spread of Covid-19 and the need for a second lockdown.

27th November

Some worrying news from the WHO reporting the outbreak of a cluster of respiratory illness in children in Northern China including severe acute respiratory syndrome coronavirus2 (SARS-CoV-2). The Chinese authorities have sought to reassure the WHO that the outbreak is limited to known pathogens but given the history of Covid-19, our health authorities would do well to remain vigilant.

Watched Andy Burnham giving evidence to the Covid-19 Inquiry. Central to his evidence was the failure of the Government in 2020 to devolve measures to the Metro Mayors and local public health authorities rather than rely on a small, ill-informed clique within Westminster. This was especially the case with 'test and trace', where local expertise in contact tracing was ignored in favour of call centres. Burnham's evidence revealed a litany of failures by the Health Minister in 2020 to communicate changes in policy to the Metro Mayors and a general disregard for their views.

30th November

Spent much of the last two days viewing Matt Hancock's evidence to the Covid-19 Inquiry. In general, he performed very well and coped with hours of forensic questioning of his role in the pandemic. Central to his interpretation of events was his view that we were three weeks late in imposing a lockdown in March 2020 and that, had the Government been more decisive and moved earlier, the level of deaths would have been a mere 10th of the subsequent fatalities. His evidence confirmed that policymaking had been increasingly compromised by the toxic atmosphere engendered by Cummings.

Once again, the Treasury and Bank of England are diverging in their assessment of our economy. While Hunt advanced an optimistic view of the UK's economic performance in his Budget Statement, the Governor of the Bank, Andrew Bailey, announced that Britain's growth potential was the worst he had seen in his lifetime and that the bank rate was likely to remain at a relatively high level for a considerable time. Moreover, while Hunt managed to introduce pre-election tax cuts without boosting borrowing, they will no doubt be paid for by implausibly tough public spending plans in future years. The Office of Budget Responsibility estimates that the measure will require austerity-style cuts in real terms of around 4% in departmental budgets.

The first snow of the winter is with us. Very scenic but hazardous and we will have to be ultra-cautious, not least because the state of the NHS is such that A&E is the last place I want to be.

8th December

An eventful week on many fronts. I managed to cope with two outings, one to the dental hygienist and one to a book group

Christmas meal at Cibo's, just outside Penicuik. Fortunately, I can still access restaurants using my smaller walker, which puts less strain on Mo when loading the car.

Worrying news from the USA where Biden has so far failed to pass his budget through Congress, without which the next tranche of military aid to Ukraine cannot be progressed. Many in the Republican Party are hostile to any open-ended commitment to Ukraine should the war continue through another winter without recourse to a negotiated settlement.

At home, Rishi Sunak has risked all by further committing the Government to the Rwanda scheme despite all the evidence that it is doomed to failure. The Rwanda (Asylum and Immigration) Bill is due to be debated next week and is increasingly viewed in the media as a vote of confidence in his premiership. The Bill is delusionary. It seeks to evade the previous ruling of the High Court against the scheme and threatens to ensure an end to legal delays by disapplying parts of the UK's Human Rights Act to asylum claims. So far, a third of a billion pounds has been invested in the scheme and not a single person has been deported. Meanwhile the recent changes to the legal immigration regulations also elevates this administration to a new level of insensitivity and inhumanity. They significantly raise the financial threshold required for skilled immigrants to obtain a visa, disallow care workers from bringing in dependants, and stipulate that British citizens or people settled in the UK must earn £38,700 before an overseas partner can join them. This will effectively deter thousands of overseas health and care workers from settling in the UK and restrict UK citizens on low incomes from bringing their partners into the country.

I have been spending a good deal of time watching the proceedings of the Covid-19 Inquiry and especially the evidence of Boris Johnson. He was clearly well briefed but his inability or unwillingness to focus on the main issues was all too evident. Throughout his evidence he framed his argument in the collective 'we' and rarely 'I'.

His recurrent mantra was that 'they' may have got things wrong from time to time but got the major decisions right. He had no convincing explanation for his absence from the COBRA meetings in February and early March of 2020, and dismissed the toxic culture of the Cabinet Office as merely the healthy clash of ideas in any policy-making institution. Similarly, he considered the marginalisation of the devolved administrations as necessary in view of their divergent political views and the advantages of a unified message given that the pandemic knew no boundaries.

Sadly, the crisis in Gaza worsens with the Israeli forces recommencing their invasion, a cessation of the exchange of hostages and prisoners, and a continuing humanitarian disaster in the few remaining areas to which the Palestinian population has been herded, devoid of heating, shelter, sustenance and medical facilities.

More details are emerging about the outbreak of pneumonia and chest infections in China in children (MPP). The WHO appears to have meekly accepted the reassurances of Chinese authorities that no new pathogen has emerged but some western paediatricians fear that MPP may be combining with Covid, or worse still mutated to a strain resistant to the only antibiotics safe for young children. As with Covid, Chinese doctors are not permitted to share information with their counterparts abroad, so we need to put pressure on the WHO to be more proactive in investigating this new threat.

16th December

The Mad Hatter's Tea Party continues unabated, and the week's news was dominated by Rishi Sunak's determination to push ahead with his ill-fated Rwanda Bill, designed to compel judges to treat Rwanda as a 'safe' country and to allow ministers to disregard sections of the Human Rights Act. He successfully navigated its Second Reading, but the likelihood is that the Bill will be severely mauled in the Lords and receive a hostile response from the Tory Right when it returns to the Commons unless it also prevents individual asylum seekers from appealing directly to the European Court of Human Rights. It is all further evidence of the lack of a moral compass in the present Westminster Government.

19th December

It is nearly four years since I started to record my experience of the Covid-19 pandemic. In many ways society has come to terms with living with the virus but its legacy of long Covid and mental illness will be profound. The Covid-19 Inquiry has in many respects been a wasted opportunity. It provided good entertainment and ruthlessly exposed the incompetence of British governance during the pandemic, but in focusing on personalities rather than processes it failed to gain real traction on the lessons to be learnt for addressing future viral threats.

As I write, the news is hugely depressing. In Ukraine, the war will be one of attrition and is likely to end in a negotiated peace that will satisfy neither side. The probability is that the USA and. NATO will soon be reining back on their military support for Ukraine under pressure from far-Right populists determined to prioritise their own national security and identity. Across Europe, there is a shift in the centre of political gravity to the Right, whether it be in France, Italy, Hungary, Sweden, Finland, or even the Netherlands, commonly informed by an anti-immigrant agenda. This shift will constrain any further promises of open-ended commitment to the Ukrainian cause.

The war in Gaza continues to produce a humanitarian disaster. It is difficult to see how the Israeli forces can destroy an ideology. The current desolation of Gaza is more likely to breed yet another generation of extremists dedicated to the elimination of the State of Israel. As with Ukraine, the prognosis is not good. At some point negotiations will have to take place, but by then there will be little infrastructure left to support the Palestinian population. Meanwhile, there is always the danger that the war will spread in the Middle East. Already, Houthi rebels, operating out of Yemen, with the support of Iran, have attacked shipping in the Suez Canal, allegedly bound for Israel, and disrupted a major artery of world trade.

A welcome distraction from the news – a flock of long-tailed tits and a blackcap on my feeders.

20th December

I had my annual consultation with the Parkinson nurse today. As always, she was very focused, and we covered a lot of ground. Interestingly, she recommended that I cease taking the extra Sinemet medication advised by my consultant. Her view was that it would be unlikely to affect my freezing and festination but merely add more side-effects. There is no sense of a unified Parkinson team in Midlothian, coordinating the work of the nurses with the neurologists. The *Movers and Shakers* podcast would suggest that this may not be the case elsewhere in the UK. The latest podcast also raised the interesting question as to whether, in the continuing absence of any significant breakthrough in finding a cure for Parkinson's, more emphasis should be placed on investing in research into more effective forms of palliative care.

30th December

A final entry after four years, most of which has been dominated by the Covid-19 pandemic and the debasement of standards in public life under the Tory Government (Typified today by the publication of Liz Truss's New Year's honours list). Apart from the development of vaccines, little has been achieved. The economy has flatlined, health and welfare services have deteriorated, and poverty has increased. The supposed benefits of Brexit have not materialised and key issues such as housing and immigration have not been properly addressed. The egregious management of the budget under the premiership of Truss, coupled with the spiralling of fuel prices, has seriously eroded the standard of living of the working and middle classes. Scottish governance under the SNP has also proved 'not fit for purpose'. Social deprivation has increased and public services such as education, health and transport have all been chronically under-funded. Instead, the focus of policymaking has been diverted to achieving Indyref2. Holyrood has also witnessed its fair share of scandals, and the financial dealings of the SNP prior to Nicola Sturgeon's resignation as First Minister are still under police investigation.

There is little evidence that the UK Government has learned any lessons from the Covid-19 Inquiry, and the massive amount of misappropriated funds expended on the provision of personal protection equipment and on support under the furlough scheme has yet to be accounted for. Meanwhile, the mental and physical damage of long Covid has not been properly acknowledged and represents a major challenge for the NHS in the future.

Sadly, the international picture is equally depressing. The wars in Sudan, Ukraine, and Israel/Gaza are all ongoing with an enormous loss of life and infrastructure and millions of displaced people. As I write, Israeli forces have renewed their destruction of Gaza in an effort to eliminate Hamas, leaving over a million

Palestinians without adequate food, water, fuel, accommodation and medical facilities. The likelihood of a resolution of the conflict is slim and the danger is that the fighting will trigger a broader, regional war. Hostilities have already begun to involve Iran-backed Shia Islamist groups in Lebanon and Yemen. In Ukraine the deadlock continues. It is likely to be prolonged and that NATO and the USA will at some point rein back on their support, especially if Donald Trump gets re-elected.

It is difficult to gauge how far I have in fact 'degenerated' over the last four years. My balance and mobility have certainly degenerated, and I am dependent on a cane or walker to move around the house, and more at risk of falling. However, there are a lot of positives. My cognitive skills are still okay. Along with my Ancestry projects, keeping this diary has enabled me to maintain my analytical and writing skills. Some memory loss but not significant. My voice is still okay, and I have no difficulty using the phone. Eyesight and perceptive skills have weakened but not to any worrying extent given that I no longer drive. Recent alterations in my medication have improved my bladder and dribbling problems and the occasional Diazepam has greatly improved my quality of life by reducing the stress of coping outwith the house. I think it is indicative of the slow deterioration in my condition that I have not yet had recourse to using my wheelchair that was purchased in April 2022. May it long continue!

www.ingramcontent.com/pod-product-compliance
Lightning Source LLC
Chambersburg PA
CBHW030327200626
46816CB00006BA/1954